The Politics of Mental Health and Illness

Series Editor
Bruce M. Z. Cohen
Sociology
University of Auckland
Auckland, New Zealand

The Politics of Mental Health and Illness conceptualises the western mental health system as a social, economic, political, and cultural project which cannot be adequately theorised without considering wider societal and structural issues such as professional power, labelling and deviance, ideological and social control, consumption, capital, and self-governance. Engaging with both social theory and empirical evidence, and situated at the intersections of critical psychiatry, sociology, anthropology, social psychology, social work, history, media studies, and the health and education sciences, the series offers academics, researchers, postgraduate students, and practitioners new and innovative monographs and edited collections with which to contest and challenge the taken-for-granted understandings of psychiatry and the mental health system currently progressed in western society. Research topics for the collection may include: aspects of the medicalisation and/or pharmaceuticalisation of everyday life; psy-professional power and knowledge production; psychopolitics and the expansion of talk therapies; the biomedical model and the future of psychiatric nosology; the marketisation of mental health discourse; social media and self-diagnosing behaviour; capitalism and psychiatric violence; and specific analyses of psy-professionals and their practices from a variety of locations (including prisons, workplaces, addiction clinics, the military, schools, the home, and general hospitals). As the first book series to explicitly encourage critical contributions in the area of mental health and illness, we welcome scholarship from a wide range of different theoretical and empirical perspectives.

If you would like to discuss a book idea prior to submitting a proposal please contact the Series Editor, Dr Bruce M. Z. Cohen, via the Commissioning Editor, Beth Farrow (beth.farrow@palgrave.com).

Janaka Jayawickrama • Jerome Wright

Under the Gaze of Global Mental Health

A Critical Reflection

palgrave
macmillan

Janaka Jayawickrama
Department of History
Shanghai University
Shanghai, China

Jerome Wright
Department of Health Sciences
University of York
York, UK

ISSN 2731-5266 ISSN 2731-5274 (electronic)
The Politics of Mental Health and Illness
ISBN 978-3-031-78257-2 ISBN 978-3-031-78258-9 (eBook)
https://doi.org/10.1007/978-3-031-78258-9

Cover illustration: Malte Mueller

This Palgrave Macmillan imprint is published by the registered company Springer Nature Switzerland AG.
The registered company address is: Gewerbestrasse 11, 6330 Cham, Switzerland

To all the individuals and communities that are suffering through uncertainty and dangers due to structural inequalities and discrimination.

Foreword

This outstanding book is a thoroughgoing and anthropologically influenced examination of the 'global mental health' (GMH) field, one with implications far beyond the primary case examples the authors use—Malawi and Sri Lanka, both largely poor non-Western states which were once part of the British Empire, but with very different cultural histories. They challenge the Western epistemology and biomedical universalism behind the definitions of 'mental health', 'wellbeing', 'stress', 'distress', increasingly used to inform programmes in non-Western settings. The GMH discourse sets out consciously to instruct, regulate, and modernise, presenting contemporary Western mentality and ways of being a person as definitive globally. When the GMH field speaks of a 'treatment gap' they wish to address worldwide, they are seeking to market the products of the Western mental health industry and its 'psy experts'.

The authors do not apply a linear, uni-disciplinary approach, but seek a holistic understanding within socio-political cultural and economic contexts of what they call the "global reality of mental health", and its expression in Malawi and Sri Lanka. This is also a critique of the colonial imposition of knowledge, assumed universal, and the displacement of time-honoured indigenous understandings of life and adversity. I have witnessed the consequences of this in my own country, Zimbabwe. As the authors quote, "in Europe they have knowledge, in Africa they have culture". Much of the GMH literature published in English-language journals fails the core test of validity, which is that methodological approaches must capture the 'nature of reality' held by subjects if they are to mean anything authentic.

As an ethical starting point, the authors emphasise that they do not claim independence, impartiality, neutrality, but that "researchers cannot be separated from the researched". Scientific objectivity is a myth: no researchers bring a blank slate and cannot but carry elements of their own background world and the culture of the educational institutions to which they have been exposed. Edward Said criticised what he called the "ritual calm" of the academic, the distancing occasioned by the supposed demands of 'objectivity'. Janaka Jayawickrama grew up in rural Sri Lanka, no stranger to extreme poverty and disaster, became a local humanitarian worker and thence journeyed through universities in the West on a social anthropology road. Jerome Wright is British, trained initially as a nurse, worked for some years in HIV before undertaking work in Malawi in both government and non-government sectors. Each has been on a journey in Western and non-Western contexts that has coloured their work.

All in all, this is an ambitious, sophisticated, and hugely engaged piece of scholarship, surely a seminal addition and corrective to so much of the published literature on GMH.

Derek Summerfield

Institute of Psychiatry
Psychology & Neuroscience
King's College London
London, UK

Acknowledgements

This book has been influenced by discussions we have had with numerous colleagues over the years. Those discussions, combined with our own research and experiences, have shaped our views on mental health and wellbeing. We would like to acknowledge Professor Karl Atkin, Dr. Bruce Cohen, and Professor David Ingleby for their encouragement in taking a different path to explore and examine the subject matter, and to the late Professor Phil O'Keefe, who helped us to locate mental health and wellbeing within a globalised capital marketplace. We offer profound gratitude to Dr. John R. Van Eenwyk and Dr. Alison Eyre for planting the seeds of critical thinking and examining mental health, especially in the Global South, and we are deeply thankful to Dr. Derek Summerfield, a mentor, collaborator, and friend for writing the foreword to this book.

We acknowledge the time and generosity of individuals and communities in Malawi, Sri Lanka, and the UK. They showed us the human capabilities to effectively deal with uncertainties and dangers of lives in disasters, conflicts, and uneven development. Without them, this book would not have become a reality.

Finally, we would like to thank our families for their patience and constant encouragements during the writing of this book.

Competing Interests We declare that there are no financial and/or non-financial interests.

Ethics The quotations that are included in this book derive from the PhD research of both Janaka Jayawickrama and Jerome Wright. There are some outside quotations that came through our lived experiences in Malawi, Sri Lanka, and the UK. We have received informed consent from the individuals within our research projects. All the individual quotations that have come through communities are presented with pseudonyms to protect their identities.

Contents

About the Authors

Janaka Jayawickrama Sri Lankan by birth and disposition, Janaka is a social anthropologist. Trained in India, the USA, and the UK, he is mostly known for his work on concepts of care, health, and wellbeing related to disasters, conflicts, and uneven development. Over the past 30 years, Janaka has been collaborating with communities in Asia, Africa, and West Asia (Middle East) in humanitarian affairs-, community development-, and wellbeing-related research and education. Janaka's research covers a range of fields. He is passionately interested in the question of how lived experiences through crises generate concepts; how we might examine philosophical traditions from Asia, Africa, Latin America, and West Asia as generative of theoretical and practical approaches to facilitate wellbeing; how to reduce the gap between human beings and nature; and how historical processes and events impact the present day and combine in the creation of purposeful critical analyses. His work on wellbeing, inclusivity, and the need for harmonious relationship with nature has appeared in many anthologies. Janaka is Professor of Anthropology and Director—Research Centre for Health and Wellbeing of the Department of History at College of Liberal Arts, Shanghai University, China. He holds many honorary positions in China, Sri Lanka, Bangladesh, Nepal, and the UK.

Jerome Wright As a registered nurse Jerome worked in a number of hospital and community health care settings in the UK, including as a nurse specialist, where he established a liaison mental health nursing service for people affected by HIV/AIDS. As a nurse and researcher Jerome has led research and community health projects in Africa and South Asia, including winning Oxfam's Susie Smith Memorial Prize for work with young people with HIV/AIDS in Malawi and examining opportunities for the integration of mental health care into non-communicable disease programmes in Bangladesh, India, and Pakistan. Jerome's PhD explored people's meanings, experiences, and responses to psychological distress in rural Malawi, with a particular interest in indigenous and traditional understandings, local expressions, and help-seeking. Jerome's work unpacks notions of 'global' mental health through critical and postcolonial perspectives that inform approaches to strengthening local health care responses. As an associate professor in the Department of Health Sciences at the University of York in the United Kingdom, Jerome collaborates with researchers, health workers and international NGOs on mental health and wellbeing initiatives across Africa, West Asia, South Asia, and Southeast Asia.

Abbreviations

ADHD	Attention Deficit Hyperactivity Disorder
AIDS	Acquired Immunodeficiency Syndrome
APIU	Acute Psychiatric In-patient Unit
COVID-19	Coronavirus Disease 2019
CMHT	Community Mental Health Team
DALY	Disability Adjusted Life Year
DSM	Diagnostic and Statistical Manual of Mental Disorders
EU	European Union
GMH	Global Mental Health
GMC	General Medical Council
GP	General Practitioner
HIV	Human Immunodeficiency Viruses
ICD	International Classification of Diseases and Related Health Problems
IMF	International Monetary Fund
JVP	Janatha Vimukthi Peramuna (People's Liberation Front)
LTTE	Liberation Tigers of Tamil Eelam
MGMH	Movement of Global Mental Health
MOMH	Medical Officer of Mental Health
NCD	Non-Communicable Diseases
NGO	Non-Governmental Organisations
PCMHC	Primary Community Mental Health Centres
PTSD	Post-Traumatic Stress Disorder
UK	United Kingdom
UN	United Nations
USA	United States of America
WB	World Bank
WHO	World Health Organisation

List of Figures

CHAPTER 1

Introduction

1.1 Approach to This Book

With this book we are attempting to establish a holistic approach to understanding the global reality of mental health and wellbeing—a reality that is shaped by social, political, cultural, economic, and environmental contexts of local realities of life in Malawi and Sri Lanka. In this, we refrain from taking a single discipline or linear analysis which flows as the mainstream epistemology from the Euro-North American context, since such an approach has a tendency to single out aspects of mental distress in a way that the rich local realities become abstract. In this too, we do not claim independence, impartiality, and neutrality, which are often seen as mainstream research principles. As researchers constructing a meaningful understanding of realities, we cannot be separated from the researched in Malawi and Sri Lanka. Indeed, there is very little justification for carrying forward any myth of scientific objectivity, particularly when the objective of our work is to bring about a change in these realities. The oppressed become strictly oppressed when they are suppressed in the mind. Our epistemic disobedience (Mignolo, 2009), of which we will narrate later, attempts to breakout from this crisis of mainstream epistemology, which has penetrated everywhere, and from which a major decolonisation of minds for everyone is required.

J. Jayawickrama, J. Wright, *Under the Gaze of Global Mental Health*, The Politics of Mental Health and Illness,
https://doi.org/10.1007/978-3-031-78258-9_1

1.2 Our Collaboration and Epistemic Injustice

If you want to go fast, go alone.
If you want to go far, go together.

A Southern African proverb

This book is a result of our journey of collaboration. This is also a journey of learning together and understanding each other. The book is an outcome of accumulative 65 years of experiences between us working on mental health, wellbeing, illnesses, disasters, conflicts, and uneven development. Janaka started as a local humanitarian worker, then became a researcher and academic. Jerome has formal training in nursing, and later became a researcher and academic. We started from different places, had diverse journeys, and ended up in the same place.

We better explain ourselves first, so we can elaborate our paths.

Janaka was born in Sri Lanka when the country was going through a transitional period. Most of his childhood was spent in rural and poor Sri Lanka where he witnessed disasters, extreme poverty, and diseases. Later, when he became a local humanitarian worker, these experiences were helpful in collaborating with conflict- and disaster-affected communities as an equal partner. His initial and foundational training comes through affected populations themselves—Sri Lanka, India, Nepal, Bangladesh, Indonesia, Kenya, Sudan, Malawi, Jordan, Iraq, and many other countries. His formal training started in 2000 with studying for a diploma in trauma treatment in the USA, which encouraged him to take up formal education. He completed an MSc in Disaster Management and Sustainable Development and a PhD in Social Anthropology in the UK, which allowed him to become an academic and researcher. As a local humanitarian worker, Janaka was exposed to Euro-North American diagnosis, and training of war trauma, post-traumatic stress disorder (PTSD), anxiety, and stress. He was disturbed that, at best, Euro-North American interventions were couched in terms of 'Do No Harm' when the reality was that many interventions were inappropriate and harming populations. For Janaka, the delivery of mental health interventions, based on individual diagnoses of PTSD was far from the service that affected populations required.

Jerome was born in the county of Suffolk in eastern England with all the apparent certainties and life prospects expected of a grammar school educated child of the 'post-war' generation. His training as a nurse in both physical and mental health specialties exposed him to a wide range of experiences of suffering and recovery. A decade working with people with

HIV/AIDS, particularly at a time when treatments were rudimentary, the prognosis very poor, and the social stigma profound and damaging, provided him key learning about both the dignity and endurance of individuals and the powerful solidarity that can be found in marginalised communities. Whilst the clinical nursing skills were sought, it was the skills of engagement and reflexivity that underpinned Jerome's first experiences working in Malawi, East Africa, with both NGO and government health services and later to leading a large community mental health task-shifting project. Here, Jerome's experiences stimulated the realisation of not only the limitations of the Western mental health 'expertise' and harm from its export, but also the potential for collaborative work to enable the promotion of existing indigenous knowledges and ways of responding to people's distress. Jerome's PhD derives from his studies examining these challenges and has developed through subsequent research work in South Asia.

We met each other in 2015, as colleagues. Through our discussions, we realised that there is a common ground between us. Jerome through his formal training in the UK and Janaka through his various learnings in many places started to engage in a dialogue. We found that this dialogue between us is an interesting one. Our positionalities are divergent, and our philosophical values extremely different. Of course, we were worried at the beginning of insulting each other's beliefs, or of offending attitudes, and closely held values. However, as we engaged through dialogue, we developed respect for each other with compassion and humility. We knew that we are never going to completely understand each other's experiences, however, we listened. In this process, we developed a deep sense of friendship and kinship, which became the foundation of our collaboration. Over the years, and in whatever shared project or independent assignment in different parts of the world, we valued the opportunity to share reflections and learning. Regardless of our differences of power through our positionalities, we found a common and equal space for us to engage.

Our collaboration is also an important element of this book. Since people from the Global North commonly go to the Global South to teach, build capacity, and conduct research, we wonder about the potential for such engagements to become friendships and equal collaborations. Our own example is that it is possible. However, the mainstream education has created an unequal space between people in the Global North and Global South. As we write this book, many capable individuals from the Global South are studying or aspiring to study in universities in Europe or North

America, so they can get 'better' education. The premise of this book is that this unequal ground must be broken. As argued by Walter Rodney (1972), Vandana Shiva (2005), Walter Mignolo (2011), and Hamid Dabashi (2015), as well as many others, it is time to break away from the colonial idea that European and North American knowledge is superior to the knowledge and wisdoms from the rest of the world. There are many different epistemologies, and they must all be treated with equal respect. We are not arguing here that Euro-North American knowledge is inferior to Asia, African, Latin America, and West Asian (Middle Eastern) knowledge. We argue rather that there must be a space for all these knowledge systems and that wisdom must be used to find solutions to the many problems we are all facing today, including health, climate crisis, and disasters.

As we suggested earlier, in many ways, this collaboration is a story of epistemic disobedience (Mignolo, 2009). We are discussing such disobedience when the world is going through some major transitions in relation to thinking. In this collaboration, we see these transitions from three different angles, and here we want to present our experiences with them.

First, the higher education institutes in the Global North are waking up to the idea of decolonising their curriculums and universities. In our experiences with these discussions on decolonisation, there are some major flaws. One of the major problems of this decolonisation discussion is that it completely ignores the fact that universities in the Global North are established to strengthen the colonial project. In that there is either no understanding or appreciation that the continuing existence of such colonial structures and systems make transformation or decolonisation impossible. Then, there is a serious lack of deeper understanding of epistemological imperialism which affects everyone in the world. Again, the decolonisation discourse in Europe and North America either ignores or seems unaware that intellectuals and scholars from the Global South have been working on decolonisation of the mind, including epistemic disobedience, as part of their independence movements. From Gandhi to Kwame Nkrumah to Frantz Fanon to Ponna Wignaraja to Walter Mignolo to Vandana Shiva are just a few examples.

As we write this book, Jerome technically sits in the Global North in Europe and Janaka technically sits in the Global South in Asia. We use the term 'technically' here with an understanding that social, economic, political, cultural, and environmental forces are shifting from the Global North to the Global South, especially from the Euro-North American context to an Asian one. Our day-to-day lives are all being affected by these shifts. This shift is also significant from the discourse of decolonising the mind and is the second angle of this transition. The foundation of modernity as we have been told and taught over the past 100 years by the Global North through a globalisation of the capital marketplace is, or at least seems to be, coming to an end. We may be wrong here. However, we understand the flip side of modernity is the colonial project that plunders, steals, and destroys many societies and populations across the globe. As we talk about epistemic disobedience, many people are waking up to question the ideals behind the modernity and development presented through capitalism.

Third, there is a generation of scholars from the Global North that are truly engaging and collaborating with the Global South. Of course, we are talking about the compassionate, caring, and humble ones here, not the 'two weeks' experts who show up in Sri Lanka or Malawi or any other country from time to time to conduct their 'research missions'. We are referring to scholars that have been working, living, and collaborating with their counterparts as equal partners. We both have been lucky enough to have learned from some of these scholars. Consciously or unconsciously, these scholars have been seeking to facilitate epistemic justice through their collaborations. As Quijano (2007) argues, there is a strong need for epistemological decolonisation to establish a clear path for new intercultural communication. We are heavily influenced by this, and we continue to practise our intercultural communication within a framework of epistemological decolonisation, which is based on compassion, care, and humility.

In this book, it is also important to explain our use of the labels Global North and Global South. Here, we are not necessarily referring to geographical locations. Global North represents the ideas of the colonial project, coloniality, modernity, and globalisation. Global South in contrast represents a response to this oppression by re-evaluating resistance, and in that, presents decolonial options of knowledge, systems, and structures. We are also aware that within North America, Australia, New Zealand, and many other settler societies (UN, 2024), there are populations that continue to be oppressed within colonial frameworks and systems. In this too, we continue to see the Global North and Global South as not geographical entities, but as a clash between oppressors and the oppressed.

In this backdrop, we are making a humble attempt to generate some ideas, thoughts, and reflections to build new groundwork for something creative and beyond the existing epistemological imperialism in mental health and wellbeing. Lewis Gordon in 'Fanon and Development: A Philosophical Look' (2004) explains this idea beyond the flawed discussions on decolonisation, and within the realities of epistemological decolonisation, and compassionate, caring, and humble intercultural communication:

> The ideas, many of which will unfold through years of engaged political work, need not be perfect, for in the end, it will be the hard, creative work of the communities that take them on. That work is the concrete manifestation of political imagination.
>
> Fanon described this goal as setting afoot a new humanity. He knew how terrifying such an effort is, for we do live in times where such a radical break appears as no less than the end of the world. In the meantime, the task of building infrastructures for something new must be planned, and where there is some room, attempted, as we all no doubt already know, because given the sociogenic dimension of the problem, we have no other option but to build the options on which the future of our species rest.
>
> Lewis Gordon, 2004
> (Cited in Mignolo, 2011, p. 44)

Within this context, our initial discussions confirmed that we were both reflecting on the Movement of Global Mental Health (MGMH) from a critical perspective. Our experiences in Malawi at different time periods and both as outsiders to the country, Janaka's work in Sri Lanka, and the fact that we were both living in the UK has given us the motivation and material to present our critique of the biomedical model of mental health within its globalising context. By no means do we argue that we are right. Actually, we may be wrong. If we knew the answers, then we would have solved the puzzle! We invite the reader to critically engage with what we present, and critically think for yourself. Here, we offer as a guide, the critical thinking and action approach proposed by Gautama the Buddha from South Asia:

> Yes, Kalamas, it is proper that you have doubt, that you have perplexity, for a doubt has arisen in a matter which doubtful. Now, look you Kalamas, do not be led by reports, or traditions, or hearsay. Be not led by the authority of religious texts, nor by mere logic or inference, not by considering

> appearances, not by the delight in speculative opinions, nor by the idea: 'this is our teacher.' But O Kalamas, when you know for yourselves that certain things are unwholesome (*akkusala*) and wrong, and bad, then give them up ... And when you know for yourselves that certain things are wholesome (*kusala*) and good, then accept them and follow them.
>
> Rahula, 1990
>
> (Cited in Henning, 2002, pp. 59–60)

1.3 Explaining Main Concepts

Throughout this book, we refer to a number of concepts such as mental health, wellbeing, conflicts, disasters, and uneven development. The meaning of some of these concepts is obvious, but some of the definitions we are using must be explained. This explanation is to establish the transparency and accountability of this book.

Mental Health: We use different definitions and concepts of mental health throughout this book. The World Health Organisation (WHO, 2022) defines mental health as a state of mental wellbeing that enables people to cope with the stresses of life, realise their abilities, learn well, and work well, and contribute to their community. At the same time, we examine mental health in connection to physical and spiritual health of individuals and communities. This idea is basically founded in an ancient definition of health. *Sushruta Samhita*, the Ayurvedic textbook of medicine and surgery (sixth century BCE) has one of the oldest definitions of health in the world: quality rest, an adequate ratio of food intake to stool output, and a harmonious relationship with society and the environment (Lad, 2002). If one is physically, mentally, and spiritually healthy, then there will only be pleasant relationships with oneself, society, and nature.

Wellbeing: Through his work over the past 30 years, Janaka defines wellbeing in disasters and conflicts against the traditional economic explanation of the concept, by defining is as the ability to live with the vagaries of life, not despite them. This is based on the idea that life is uncertain and dangerous, and it is human to deal with them. This definition has already influenced global humanitarian structures, especially in collaborations with affected populations on the ground.

> Dangers and uncertainties are an inescapable dimension of life and wellbeing is the competence to live with uncertainty. Unpredictability makes life

> fulfilling, as it is part of human nature to deal with it. … The idea here is simply to point out that, though not knowing some things can create frustration, anger and helplessness, a process of pragmatic engagement with uncertainty can create a sense of wellbeing.
>
> Jayawickrama (2008, p. 2)

Conflicts: Conflict can be defined as a clash between individuals, communities, and countries, arising out of a difference in thought process, attitudes, understanding, interests, requirements, and even sometimes perceptions.

Disasters: According to O'Keefe et al. (1976), when human systems affect the natural processes, they become disasters. For example, an earthquake only becomes a disaster when human beings, properties, and structures are affected.

Uneven Development: A term used to represent the process by which capitalism transforms the world as a whole but does so in different ways, developing the productive and social forces in some areas, but (as part of the same process) restricting or distorting growth in others (Smith & O'Keefe, 1980).

Global Mental Health (GMH): A term used to denote moves to expand biomedical notions of mental health and wellbeing through the medicalising or 'psychiatrising' of the experience of distress. Central to its aim is the reduction of the 'treatment gap' which is indicated by subtracting the availability of 'effective' interventions for the treatment of mental and neurological conditions from evidence of epidemiological studies and estimates of these disorders. Contained within this mission are universal assumptions about the understanding, experience, and treatment of mental health problems.

Movement for Global Mental Health (MGMH): refers to activity deriving a specific call for the advancement of GMH by the Lancet Global Mental Health Group (2007) through systematic research and implementation techniques and using epidemiological, behaviour change, education, and evaluation modalities. Although the MGMH can be seen to include an amalgam of organisations committed to the advancement of GMH, we use the term when referring to specific initiatives and projects that seek the same aims.

1.4 Understanding the Case Studies

The two case studies we are using in this book are from Malawi and Sri Lanka. As mentioned, we have connections to these locations, and value our experiences for various reasons. For Janaka, Sri Lanka is home, and he has been working there since 1994 in different capacities. For both Jerome and Janaka, Malawi is a place we have worked and have fond memories, friendships, and most importantly, it is the place we have learned about people, culture, and mental health.

Located in Southern Africa, Malawi, shares its borders with Mozambique, Zambia, and Tanzania (see Fig. 1.1). The country's estimated population is 20.41 million (2022) with a rapidly growing population, which has been identified as one of the complex drivers of poverty. According to the Malawi National Human Development Report (UNDP, 2021), this creates challenges to the provision of services, which include health, education, environment protection, and natural resources. The majority of the population in Malawi is highly dependent on a subsistence economy. From time to time, Malawi hits global news headlines as a place of chronic poverty, droughts, and famines. The name Malawi may have originated from the word Maravi, which was part of the Maravi Empire. According to people in Malawi, the Maravi Empire was founded in the late fifteenth century by Amaravi people who eventually became known as the Chewa. Prior to their contact with Portuguese colonisers, the Empire was prosperous and successful in maintaining the health and wellbeing of their people. However, the Empire started to decline due to invasions by Ngoni and Yao people as well as by Arabs prior to the appearance of Europeans. The Portuguese were reportedly the first Europeans to arrive in Malawi in about 1859. From 1883 until the independence in 1964, Malawi was under various forms of domination from the British Empire. The British colonial government opened the Zomba Lunatic Asylum in the southern region in 1910.

Sri Lanka is an island state in the Indian Ocean and is separated from peninsular India by the Palk Strait (see Fig. 1.2). Proximity to the Indian subcontinent has facilitated close cultural interaction between Sri Lanka and India from ancient times. Sri Lanka gained independence from Britain in 1948, and has since experienced patches of conflicts in 1971, 1987–1989,

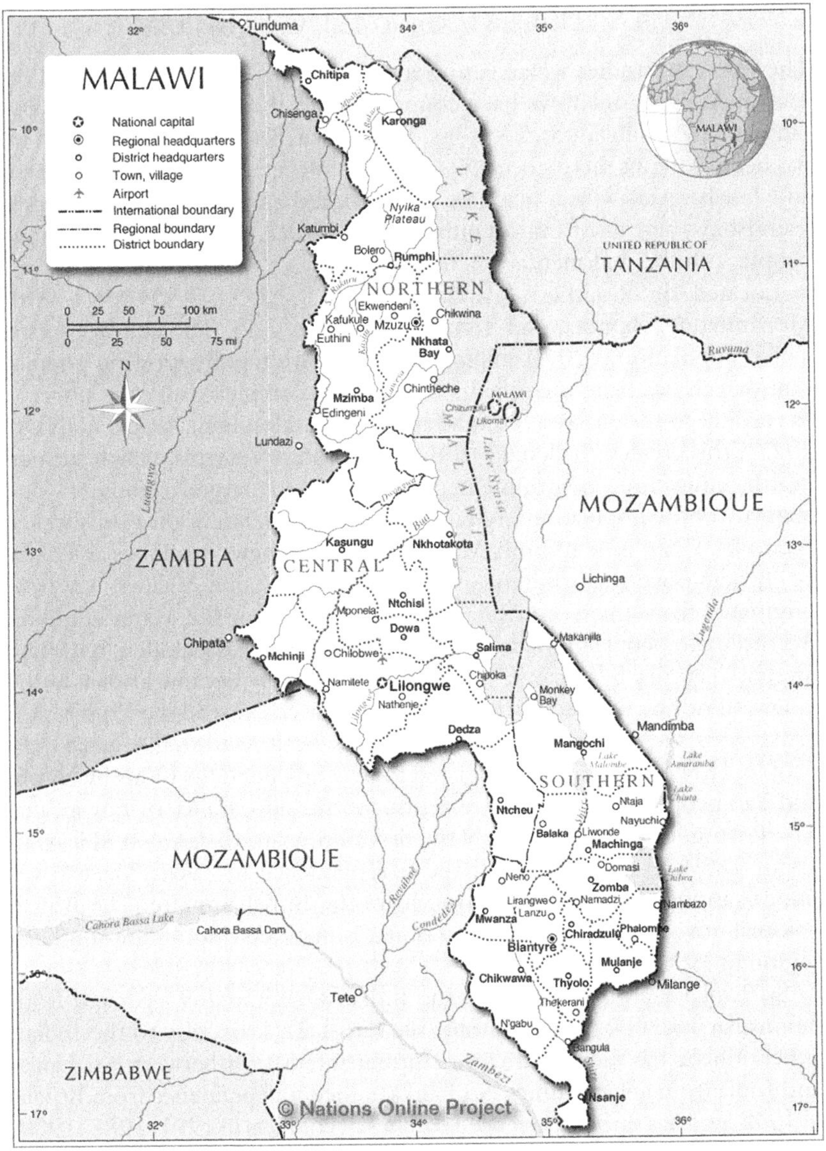

Fig. 1.1 Map of Malawi. (Source: One World—Nations Online, OWNO, nationsonline.org)

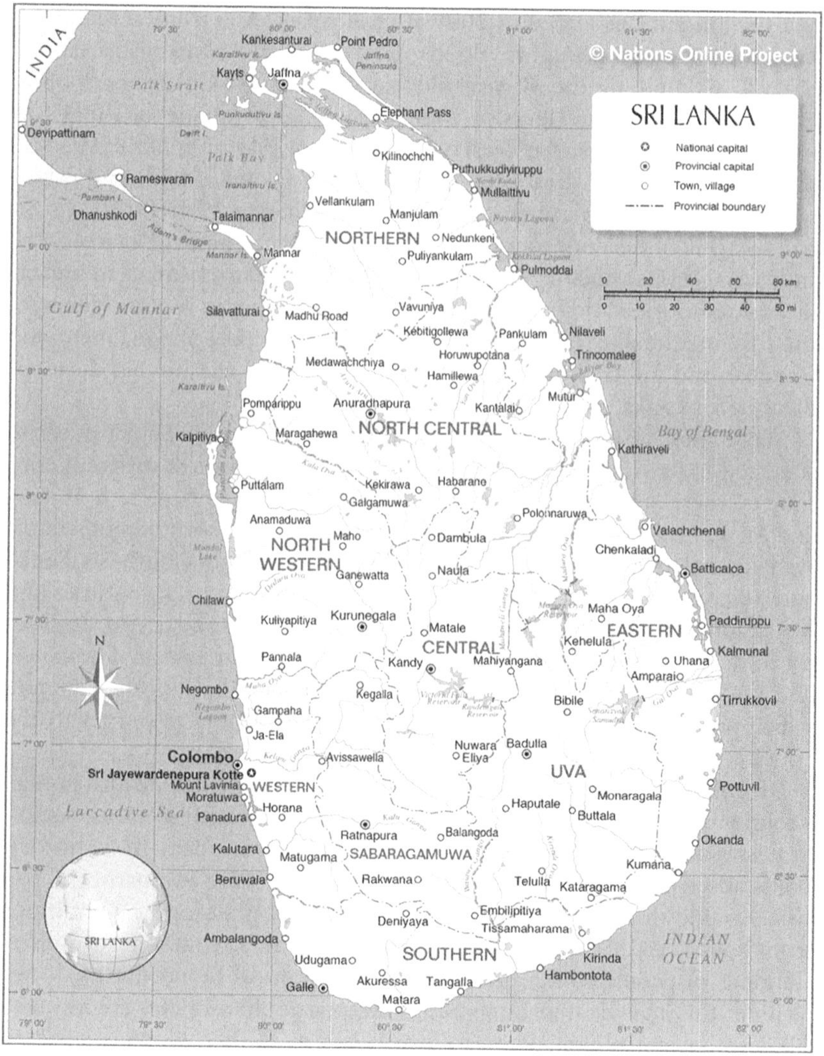

Fig. 1.2 Map of Sri Lanka. (Source: One World—Nations Online, OWNO, nationsonline.org)

and the longest one ended in 2009 after 30 years. As a tropical island, Sri Lanka experiences droughts, floods, landslides, and tsunamis as natural hazards. Combining the 30-year-old war between the Government of Sri Lanka and Liberation Tigers of Tamil Eelam (LTTE) with the 2004 tsunami disaster, Sri Lanka has been one of the many pilot sites of the MGMH over the years. The country has a 22.8 million people (2023) and is currently going through a financial crisis. According to UNDP (2021), Sri Lanka is one of the countries that performed well in Human Development Indicators (HDI) since 1990. This was due to early investments in universal basic education and basic health care. However, more recent challenges such as inequitable economic development, regional inequalities, and irregular and informal employment, have impacted the human development in Sri Lanka.

While these case studies have many differences, with Sri Lanka an island state and Malawi a landlocked country, and their location in different continents, there are several key similarities. The UK colonised both Malawi and Sri Lanka, and both countries generally function with administrative systems that derive from the colonial era. Similarly, too, both Sri Lanka and Malawi have traditional medical approaches going back centuries and which function today with varying degrees of visibility and access. And yet for both countries, the biomedical model of health care system dominates, and both countries are going through economic and political challenges which present parallels in developing their own cultural responses to the construction of mental health and wellbeing.

To compare these two case examples, we have taken ideas from a human geography perspective as well as the disciplines of health sciences, sociology, and anthropology. Further, we have drawn on ideas from history, political sciences, and economics in constructing these comparisons. You will also find that we have borrowed from ancient philosophical traditions from South Asia, Southern Africa, and Europe to strengthen our understanding of people's life experiences and responses. By no means do we claim in this analysis that Euro-North American philosophies are less useful, and ancient philosophies are much better. Rather, we have tried to respect people's contexts and learning and to take what is useful without discriminating between philosophical traditions.

1.5 The Structure of This Book

The book is structured into chapters that describe the journey of our thinking about GMH, MGMH and mental health and wellbeing from conceptual origins to their operationalisation in our two case examples.

This first chapter has introduced the personal and professional positionalities of the authors to provide the reader with important contextual detail from which our assertions are made. We also defined some recurrent terms that we will be referring to repeatedly in the book and have introduced the reader to some essential background about each of our case example countries.

Chapter 2 explores the origin and nature of stress and distress, the plurality of understandings from different settings and how the illness model deriving from the European/North American template has become the focus of global health concern. The advancing medicalisation and the growth of psy-experts is plotted alongside the links of stress and distress within political and socio-economic conditions.

Chapter 3 extends the understanding of GMH concerns through an historical analysis of the imposition of knowledge through colonialism. A brief contextual history of colonial psychiatry is offered, followed by more detailed descriptions of experiences in Malawi and in Sri Lanka, of how existing local helping and healing traditions are ignored, denigrated, and side-lined by GMH advancement.

In Chap. 4, this analysis is developed further by looking behind what is espoused in MGMH initiatives in an exploration of the responses of people to the perceived limitations and inadequacies of response to people's suffering. Case examples from the two countries are offered where local health workers resist the confines of the biomedical approach and create opportunities for healing that are plausible to the people they serve.

Chapter 5 reviews the ideas of colonialism and coloniality from the context of the UK as the colonising power. As the boomerang theory (Césaire, 2000) indicates, we offer a critical reflection on the impacts of inequalities and hierarchies of power on the UK mental health hegemony and discover responses and reactions that mirror those from Malawi and Sri Lanka. A mass casualty event from the UK's recent past, with its impact on the surviving community, provides an emphasis on the importance of community-based values and needs that can be obscured by GMH imaginings of distress.

Chapter 6 seeks to develop the appreciation of the impact of colonialism and its continued influence through coloniality and globalisation towards a discussion of alternative approaches to people's distress. The analysis of capitalist neoliberal agendas and their damage to human relations and health is the backdrop for some approaches that are emerging beyond the GMH approach and empirically testing social responses that engage local communities' knowledges and resources. A collaborative framework is offered to guide the efforts of insider and outsider partners to facilitate practical, credible, and sustained responses.

Chapter 7 brings together a summary of the book's main arguments; from insights into the dominant nature of GMH and its epistemic injustices brought to existing and ancient wisdoms, to reflections on the need for strengthening social and community-based responses. Such insights and actions denote a de-colonising of the mind whereby an appreciation of the plurality of understandings and range of expertise from both insiders and outsiders is coupled with a recognition of the need to place the responses in the hands of the communities affected and to establish collaborative partnerships of equals in strengthening people's mental health and wellbeing.

There is no one history, account, or analysis, of phenomena as broad as how people experience and manage distress. There are always alternative understandings and interpretations, and these chapters represent our learning and reflections on our experiences navigating the response to distress and distressing circumstances at a time when the MGMH and the overall hegemony of GMH was first being impressed on the world. We are interested in how different peoples experience and react to these advances, and in so doing we encounter medical, social, cultural, and political theory that help us to understand these experiences. This is therefore not primarily a theoretical discussion but is rather a reflection on experiences—both ours and of others. At best it is a recognition of theory that derives from experience that has emerged from our own learning and mistakes—and hope that in the end we offer ideas from which others can develop meaningful and practical ways to respond to the challenge of promoting mental health and wellbeing for us all.

References

Césaire, A. (2000). *Discourse on colonialism* (J. Pinkham, Trans.). Monthly Review Press.

Dabashi, H. (2015). *Can non-Europeans think?* Bloomsbury Publishing.

Henning, D. H. (2002). *A manual for Buddhism and deep ecology* (Special Ed.). The World Buddhist University.
Jayawickrama, J. (2008). *Why is there more laughter in refugee camps than on the streets of London?* Royal Geographical Society / Institute of British Geographers.
Lad, V. (2002). *Textbook of Ayurveda: Fundamental principles of Ayurveda.* Ayurvedic Press.
Lancet Global Mental Health Group. (2007). Scale up services for mental disorders: A call for action. *The Lancet, 370*, 1241–1252.
Mignolo, W. D. (2009). Epistemic disobedience, independent thought and decolonial freedom. *Theory, Culture & Society, 26*(7–8), 159–181.
Mignolo, W. D. (2011). Geopolitics of sensing and knowing: On (de) coloniality, border thinking and epistemic disobedience. *Postcolonial Studies, 14*(3), 273–283.
O'Keefe, P., Westgate, K., & Wisner, B. (1976). Taking the naturalness out of natural disasters. *Nature, 260*(5552), 566–567.
Quijano, A. (2007). Coloniality and modernity/rationality. *Cultural Studies, 21*(2–3), 168–178.
Rodney, W. (1972). Problems of third world development. *Ufahamu: A Journal of African Studies, 3*(2), 27–47.
Shiva, V. (2005). *Earth democracy: Justice, sustainability and peace.* Zed Books.
Smith, N., & O'Keefe, P. (1980). Geography, Marx, and the concept of nature. *Antipode, 12*(2), 30–39.
The Government of Malawi. (2021). *Malawi National Human Development Report 2021.* United Nations Development Programme.
United Nations. (2024). *Non-self-governing territories.* The United Nations and Decolonization.
WHO. (2022). *Mental health key facts.* Mental health Fact Sheet. https://www.who.int/news-room/fact-sheets/detail/mental-health-strengthening-our-response

CHAPTER 2

Stress and Distress as Global Health Concerns

2.1 Distress as the Cost of 'Living'

Nature has nothing to offer me that does not give rise to doubt and anxiety.
Blaise Pascal (1623–1662)
(From Pascal, 2008, p. 80)

Pascal's reflection on the nature of life and living can be seen as at the same time both reassuring and unsettling. In defining stress as "a natural human response that prompts us to address challenges and threats in our lives", the World Health Organisation (2023) similarly supposes coping with stress as an inevitable accompaniment to human existence. Scholars such as Jayawickrama (2008) and Kleinman (2006) argue that with a life full of uncertainties and stressful events, dealing with them is part of being human, and results naturally in the experience of distress. According to Hindu and Buddhist traditions too, suffering is central to human life, because everything in this world lacks permanent existence (Henning, 2002; Radhakrishnan, 1950, 1963).

By foregrounding such truths within our understandings of 'stress' and 'distress', this chapter approaches its analysis of the place of biomedicine in responding to people's distress, not in a way that repeats the comprehensive and compelling critical analysis offered by previous critical mental

J. Jayawickrama, J. Wright, *Under the Gaze of Global Mental Health*, The Politics of Mental Health and Illness,
https://doi.org/10.1007/978-3-031-78258-9_2

health scholars such as Kleinman (1977), Summerfield (2008), Fernando (2014), Mills (2014), Cohen (2016), Brossard and Chandler (2022), but rather to provide an account that is centred on the experiences of people reacting to their lives and life events within their personal, community, political and socio-cultural contexts. We will explore the influence of the medicalisation of distress; its link to capitalism and marketplace economics, its socially constructed origins and operationalisation and its function to individualise and de-politicise its impacts. In this we see people's attempts to understand and navigate towards a resolution to their distress as inseparable from these powerful contextual forces.

The emergence of Euro-North American medicalised thinking from post-enlightenment onwards has brought less tolerance that human reactions to the uncertainties and stresses of life are seen as normal. Conrad and Bergey (2015) define medicalisation as the practice where nonmedical problems become defined as disease or illness requiring medical treatment. Within the discourse of medicalisation, aspects of rage and frustration towards living conditions, and experiences of loss all become mental health problems that require medical treatment. Not only this, but the very operationalisation of biomedicine may be seen as operating in contradiction to understandings of natural processes such as birth, growth, and dying. From one perspective, humans are a part of nature and subject to natural processes, and yet from another perspective, nature is understood to be external to humans. Such difference of thinking—and understanding of fundamental notions—exemplifies that mainstream scientific approaches to health are not universal. This is especially clear when it comes to people's knowledge of health and wellbeing from Africa, Asia, and Latin/South America, as well as the indigenous philosophies from North America, Australia, and New Zealand, where, for instance, separations of mind from body are seldom made. Such differences distinguish a 'global' knowledge from 'local' knowledge and with it frequently introduce contested notions of national identity and modernity (Del Casino, 2004). Indeed, scholars such as Carrozza (2015) and Funtowicz and Ravetz (1993) have warned against the predisposition towards giving sciences and scientists an exclusive role in health and social policymaking while disregarding the wisdoms of laypeople.

2.2 The Continuities of Biomedical Universalism

Medicalisation can also be seen to have extended to the realm of economic related challenges with uneven development and poverty now becoming linked to mental illness, and since economic and financial structures are an integral part of modern societies, when these fail, people face many challenges. For example, when the 2007 economic recession began, the European Commission (2013) reported that almost half of the citizens knew someone who had lost their job as a direct consequence of the crisis. In Sri Lanka, it was reported that lower levels of education, asset ownership, and living in deprived areas were associated with an increased risk of suicidal behaviour among men and women (Knipe et al., 2019). In Malawi, with huge uneven development conditions, Jumbe et al. (2022) report that socio-economic conditions are strongly associated with mental health problems among youth. Frasquilho et al. (2015) have concluded that economic and financial challenges are associated with a high prevalence of mental health problems, including common mental disorders, substance disorders, and ultimately suicidal behaviour. Such terms and associated assumptions represent the medicalisation of responses to the stresses of life and commodification of the "mind" through professional expert endorsement. Within such hegemony, the media too, play a key role in asserting the language of psychological deficit within the imagination of the public, so that when people are experiencing socio-economic and environmental hardship, they come to see themselves not simply as dealing with the uncertainty and dangers of life, but as themselves "distressed" and "ill" with mental health problems.

However, there is no doubt that life brings stresses. Whether one lives in a 'developed' or 'developing' country and are going through difficult socio-economic, experiences, everyone faces a variety of distresses in life. A young father in a European country loses his job due to the COVID-19 pandemic and goes through a painful divorce. A young woman in an African country finds out that she has HIV. A seemingly happy family in the USA is mourning their son's suicide and the mother seeks solace in alcohol and family relationships fracture. Beyond these types of uncertainties, the economic recessions, job losses, rising house bills, unexpected health crises, and even road accidents impact on people. Even situations that look stable can bring distress into life. Modern societies are fast-paced and resource heavy. To maintain a stable lifestyle, people are increasingly pushed to work harder and harder. Contrary to the mainstream belief that hard work is equal to success, the reality frequently tells a different story. Finding an affordable home in a major city close to work can be impossible, and can result in people having a long and exhausting commutes. This takes away from family time, leisure, and social interactions, which are the very resources required to deal with distress. Despite the long hours, many jobs in contemporary societies become victim to changing markets and have limited security. Such precariousness of jobs results in heightened competition between employees, driving distrust and creating disharmony in the workplace. Despite maintaining this stressful hard work, many people find that their salaries are insufficient to take care of themselves and their families.

Ironically, or perhaps by design within complex economies, the exertion of power that creates such inequalities and occupational and economic helplessness continues to purport notions of individual worth and responsibility through expanded conceptions of 'mental health' and mental health problems. The fragmentation of societies, disorientation of individuals and families, alienation, irrational beliefs, and precarious thinking are mostly attributed to stress and distress generated within socio-economic and cultural, structures and all these conditions create sadness, frustration, fear, and anger. Here, the medical model explains these as conditions that need to be medically treated and this medicalisation of stress distracts attention away from social struggles. Purpose in life is replaced with diagnoses. So, given this background, what is meant when we describe a person as being stressed or distressed, and how are such experiences understood? What individual and population level mechanisms have been used to provide explanations for these experiences and how are these linked to medicalised notions of difference, deviance, or mental disorder?

2.3 The Social Construction of Distress

While over recent decades many theorists have espoused the contribution of 'moderate' stress or even '*eustress*' (positive stress) to individuals' optimal functioning, growth and creativity, the impact of severe external pressures or life events (be they acute threats or ongoing everyday hassles) on peoples' ability to function and survive has been evidenced by profound psychological and physical effects (Holmes & Rahe, 1967; Rabkin & Struening, 1976; Leventhal & Ian, 2012). Such a model of stress exposes all of us to the notion that given a set of circumstances any of us risk feeling overwhelmed whereby the demands of the stressful events exceed our abilities to cope. This exchange between external threats and a person's internal thought processes on their ability to respond to the stressor is seen as central to whether a person's stress becomes overwhelming and turns to 'distress'. While primarily seen as a psychological or cognitive process, such a depiction also resurrects the action of 'homeostasis' originally coined by Walter B. Cannon in 1932 and derived from Darwinian terms in which stress is seen as an internal failure of the organism to adapt to changing environmental conditions and achieve homeostasis. In his book, the Age of Stress, Mark Jackson (2013) explores the evolution of such thinking, explaining that stress has both environmental and socioeconomic conditions AND psychological and emotional concepts. Indeed, according to Jackson, stress is regarded as an endemic disease of post-industrial capitalist societies, a condition that owed its prevalence to the 'chronic strains of life'.

The idea of the need to retain an 'equilibrium' resonates across biological and social understandings. Research has attempted to develop an appreciation of how such a homeostatic process might be moderated through both individual biological and genetic variables and wider sociocultural influences (e.g., Hans Seyle's 'general adaptation syndrome'). But whatever, this emphasis of individual susceptibility and early experiences has steered towards a focus on individuation and the medicalisation of distress. Thus, distress or suffering can encompass a range of experiences, from worried thoughts, pre-occupations, ruminations, self-doubt, low mood to an existential crisis of not wishing to remain alive. Such an experience often leads to attempts to mitigate or resolve these uncomfortable feelings through behaviours such as use of drugs, alcohol, or different forms of self-harm, which can in turn lead to a spiralling descent and difficulty emerging from this distress. All societies link this kind of distress to different conceptions of suffering that occur without physical explanation, that is, mental distress or 'madness' of some kind. And yet while all societies possess notions of normality and health, the constructs of mental illness that derive are a product of definitions of social behaviour unique to the local historical and cultural understandings (Helman, 2007 p. 246). Helman identified that societies' perceptions of certain behaviours can be defined within four possible categories or 'zones'; as 'normal', accepted behaviour (controlled normality), as 'bad' or criminal where a person is aware of rules but breaks them (uncontrolled normality), as abnormal behaviour but acceptable in specific occasions or contexts such as religious states, at certain rituals or festivities (controlled abnormality) and as 'mad' within that society (uncontrolled abnormality). It's clear therefore that defining normality from abnormality varies between cultures, in that while certain behaviour may be accepted in one culture, it is not necessarily acceptable elsewhere.

Of course, from such a society's perspective, what is also apparent is that within each 'zone' society recognises a spectrum of behaviour. People committing parking violations, for instance, tend not to carry the same perspective as those who have murdered, and in a similar way, madness too often carries with it different perceptions of severity. Yet it's also clear that the four zones themselves expand and contract when comparing between and even within societies. Certainly, medicalisation brings with it an expansion of the 'madness' zone.

It's also clear that these 'zones' are fluid and subject to change over time, such as between generations or, in certain circumstances, as a reaction to external pressures or threats. Examples of this include alcohol and drug-taking, sexuality, and customs of marriage or divorce, religious conviction, or affiliation. Nevertheless, whatever the context, such labelling of abnormal and uncontrolled behaviour demonstrates the social construction of 'madness'—a labelling that endorses a particular identity and expectation towards seeking help to return to 'normal'. A person's individual perception of their own behaviour may of course be at odds with society's view (for many, this is the very definition of madness) and resisted (to avoid a stigmatised identity), and yet this can also be more evenly contested in less severe presentations of distress. Older people in the UK, for instance, may acknowledge to close family that they may be struggling or feeling low in mood but vehemently reject a GP's diagnosis of depression (UMDS MSc in General Practice Teaching Group, 1999). Specific medical or psychiatric terms therefore can be seen as carrying with them particular meaning and certain cultural and lifestyle norms and values that may of course be alien to local context. So, for instance, in Malawi, tracing the borderland between normality and 'pathology', madness is illustrated by the term *kukumudwe* (seen as a severe yet sane reaction to life's hardships) as against '*nkhawa*' (low mood /despair) which remains sane, but verging towards a pre-cursor to *misala* or madness (Wright & Maliwichi-Senganimalunje, 2020). Most people experiencing *kukamudwe* or indeed *nkhawa* do not become 'insane', but both are logically seen as implicated in the mechanism that can lead to *misala*. In other words, this may represent one (social) explanation for the 'madness', alongside other attributions that may or may not include spiritual, supernatural, or biological causes. Such subtle shifts of language represent the refining and culturally shaping of conceptions of normality and abnormality.

In Sri Lanka, the common Sinhala (one of the main languages) term for daily stressors to madness is *Pissu* (පිස්සු). One could use this term for the stressors of everyday challenges as well as insane behaviour. In this, the technical terms such as distress, stress, or depression are not in common Sinhala language. During the 30-year-old war, the 1987–1989 unrest in the Southern part of Sri Lanka, as well as the 2004 tsunami, brought many International NGOs, researchers, and various experts to work on the mental health of the population. Of course, people were suffering from emotional distress due to conflicts, disasters, and uneven development challenges. However, the question was and is whether or when this is best labelled as mental disorders, and whether individual clinical help (based on models developed in Euro-North American context) should be offered as the solution (Argenti-Pillen, 2003).

2.4 Biomedical Attributions and Their Critiques

A long history of research into these social constructions of mental health and illness expose different experiences of mental distress, conceptions of 'madness' and explanatory models of mental disorder and help-seeking through folk, popular, professional sectors in different societies and cultures (Kleinman, 1980; Kleinman & Good, 1985; Littlewood & Lipsedge, 1997; Cohen et al., 2016) revealing a huge pluralism. Causal explanations derive from physical, biological, social, psychological, and spiritual or supernatural domains, many accepted concurrently. Identifying psychopathology ("a psychological state without normal functioning requiring treatment" Stevenson, 2010, p. 190) is also ubiquitous in societies—and is not restricted to biomedical explanations. Understandings from traditional communities throughout the world have sophisticated constructions and interpretations of people's distress with, for instance, much of an African Traditional Healer's work centred on identifying (diagnosing) the cause or culprit before recommending treatments (Steinforth, 2009).

Nevertheless, the biomedical attribution or explanation of mental illness dominates international and national mental health programmes through the prominence of biomedical health care training and provision. Here, a health professional's determining that an experience of distress has become an illness—or mental disorder—is governed by the two biomedical classification systems of Diagnostic Statistical Manual (DSM) (American Psychiatric Association, 2013) and International Classification of Diseases (ICD) (WHO, 2022). And yet such taxonomies of discrete illnesses place psychiatric diagnoses apart from all other biomedical diagnoses where biological markers or bodily changes indicate its presence. Despite decades of investment into the neuroscience of mental illnesses, no biological causative links have been established (Horwitz, 2003). Indeed, the failure of biomedical science to illicit pathological markers that isolate any mental 'diseases' is seen by many to test the very scientific basis of psychiatry. The use of psychiatric diagnoses, the limitations of therapeutic effectiveness (Sartorius et al., 1986), and the 'individualising' of communal distress all highlight the precarious basis on which to frame mental distress when a biomedical approach is used to define particular 'life problems' as mental health problems (Fernando, 2014; Bentall, 2010; Moncrieff, 2009; Summerfield, 2008).

Identifying the same 'symptom' of a particular mental 'disorder' in two distinct settings does not mean that both carry the same understanding, experience, or meaning. Proposing one medicalised worldview through which to view these experiences risks a 'categorical fallacy' (Kleinman, 1977; Clark, 2014) whereby cross-cultural reliability and validity are questioned. This over-reliance on a concern for measurement and diagnosis rather than the social and cultural context is seen by many as resulting in a narrow and exclusive determining of distress (White & Sashidharan, 2014).

Indeed, the universalistic assumptions implicit in the biomedical approach to mental illness would be less contested if the evidence for the effectiveness of such approaches was more compelling. Initial and long-term follow-up studies from the 1970s showed superior rates of recovery in many low-resource countries, when compared to Western countries (Sartorius et al., 1986). This questioned the appropriateness of offering psychotropic medication, with all its iatrogenic effects, and Western-premised 'talking treatments' where there is no evidence of local effectiveness (Moncrieff, 2009; Bentall, 2010; Summerfield, 2008; Kirmayer, 2012).

By medicalising and individualising a person's distress, and diverging from the many communal ways of understanding the nature, causes, and effects of peoples' distress, also diverts attention away from the socio-economic and political environments like poverty, violence, inequality, and discrimination that have been shown to cause such distress (Allen & Feigl, 2017). As a result, structural social determinants of distress are submerged by the development of individualised therapeutic interventions (Saxena et al., 2006) and consequently risks and causes become de-politicised (Mills & Fernando, 2014). Jackson (2013) himself worries that such a medicalised focus on individual (biological) mechanisms of distress risks limiting attention to socio-economic factors ('stressors' in Seyle's terminology) in the incidence of stress-related diseases, such as obesity and heart disease, and the very real health challenges it presents particularly for the poor and underprivileged.

Yet the hegemony of distress as an individualised problem dominates the discourse in most of the Global North. Among countless examples is a recent survey commissioned by the UK's Mental Health Foundation (2023). Launched in response to 'cost of living' concerns and increasing poverty deriving from the post-COVID-19 pandemic and the war in Ukraine (and following the UK government's decade of economic austerity policies), the study asked 3000 adults about their mental health. Perhaps unsurprisingly, more than one-third (34%) felt anxious and one in ten (10%) of UK adults felt hopeless about financial circumstances. And yet the report seamlessly goes on to define the individual experience of stress and advise on how individuals can 'cope' with advice on 'how you can help yourself'.

In a similar way, a recent process evaluation of non-communicable disease (NCD) clinics in Bangladesh and Pakistan to investigate the opportunities to introduce psychological intervention for attendees with depression revealed that the source of distress was not the actual NCD or even any worsening symptoms, but more the frustrations over lack of resources to attend appointments, and the availability and affordability of medications (Wright et al., 2020).

Of course, within this critique there is always the danger that in challenging individualisation and the medicalising of distress, the genuine suffering becomes overlooked or secondary to some academic or esoteric discussion. In both examples—from the UK and from Bangladesh and Pakistan—there is no doubt that people are distressed, with all the personal, familial, community and wider societal impact that this has. But by adopting a medicalising and individualising position, its resolution assumes an individual rather than a social change and the removal of structural barriers or deficits.

The study in Bangladesh and Pakistan also highlights the effects of using the language of biomedicine or psychiatry within different environments (Wright et al., 2020). While individual suffering clearly existed, patients were not familiar with describing this under a label of 'depression' or of some kind of mental deficiency or illness. Such positioning places individuals' mental health within a marketplace of the 'demand' and 'supply' elements of the mental health treatment gap (WHO, 2013), attracting powerful avocations for both mental health literacy and evidenced mental health interventions (Fernando, 2014; Patel & Prince, 2010). With its unapologetically grounded biomedical thinking and accompanying epidemiological research based on estimates of the global burden of disability (Kohn et al., 2004), the global mental health agenda has drawn attention to the needs of 'vulnerable' populations and has used human rights-based rhetoric to inspire action at government and intergovernmental levels through a series of action plans and intervention guides (WHO, 2013, 2016). Increasing the supply of biomedical mental health provision is now asserted across primary care provision (Lund et al., 2015).

And yet this logic of response to a growing pandemic of mental health problems advocated by surveys of Disability Adjusted Life Year (DALYs) measures can be contested not by rejecting the reality of people's distress but by demonstrating changes to how such distress is perceived. In a striking study challenging the assumed unremitting worldwide rise in distress, Amy Johnson (2021) compared the US national health interview survey data across 20 years. Her findings identified no change in levels of distress within the population but did show a significant increase in help-seeking. Johnson's conclusion, that "individuals' mental health behaviours are responding to changing context over time even if their subjective mental health is not" (p. 63) clearly implicates the socio-cultural evidence of labelling theory to illustrate this diversity in the experience of distress. Such findings emphasise further Brossard and Chandler's (2022) correction to the assumptions drawn from the epidemiological evidence of DALYs by instead arguing a subtle and more precise observation—that whatever its origin, explanation or standpoint, and ever widening sphere of influence, "the mental health crisis indicates: that serious amounts of people claim to experience behavioural troubles and emotional distress, and that an impressive web of institutions and services … is deployed to monitor, define and respond to their suffering" (p. 119).

Thus, despite the medicalised hegemony and prominent political rhetoric where 'common mental disorders' have even been subsumed into the global Sustainable Development Goals (Votruba & Thornicroft, 2016), a closer examination reveals that distress, and its responses need to be understood within the overall health of an individual, and individual health is located within the social, political, cultural, economic, and environmental context in which they live.

However, what we may forget is that mainstream science is itself socially constructed—what we study, the questions we ask, the approaches we accept or reject. Contrary to the mainstream idea, science and scientists sit within, not outside, society. And capitalism, as advanced by the Global North is the dominant frame through which this is realised, with its emphasis on expanding markets, consumers, and profit. Is it a surprise that distress and mental health problems are absorbed within this same frame?

In 2023, a report by the marketing firm Prophecy Market Insights (2023) estimated that by 2030 the global mental health market will reach US$ 527.44 billion. The analysis goes on to anticipate that this market will expand "as a result of increased education about mental diseases, advocacy work for more human rights respect, and efforts to reduce stigma" (Prophecy Market Insights, 2023). Seeking profit from suffering is one thing, but an acknowledgement that approaches to health education and even human rights advocacy work are marketing opportunities places mental health fully within a particular socio-cultural context. The fact that this bio-medicalised approach to mental health problems originates from Europe and North America is by no means a coincidence. The hegemonic control employed by such medicalising agendas, whereby self-surveillance, self-care and treatments are promoted to summon an individual's 'mental health', is a profitable enterprise—underpinned by global markets, consumerism, and big pharma (Cohen, 2016). Indeed, the pharmaceutical industry's links with psychiatry appear to extend to the very body that defines mental disorder. According to Pilecki et al. (2011) approximately 70% of the task force members devising the DSM-V reported financial relationships with the pharmaceutical industry. Mental illness and capitalism thus appear intrinsically bound, and this medicalising process is situated as the continuance of a long-term endeavour starting at least a century earlier in European history. Understanding the historical-socio-political-economic context of colonialism can help to appreciate the ways in which concepts of mental health have aligned with the dominant discourse of the powerful and that have been enacted to this day.

2.5 Coloniality and Control

Our case studies in this book are both affected by the colonial project. Between 1505 and 1948 Sri Lanka was colonised by first the Portuguese, and then the Dutch, and British. According to McCracken (2012), Malawi was "discovered" by the Portuguese, and in 1859 David Livingstone "discovered" Lake Malawi, and so between 1883 and 1964, Malawi was colonised by the British. Links between medicalised understandings of mental illness and racism can be traced to these early interactions with people in such colonies. Davis (2018) has pointed towards the immunity hypothesis, which claimed that enslaved Africans were seen in the early nineteenth century as immune to mental illness. He argues that this connects psychiatry to politics rather than to slaves' experience of mental health and wellbeing:

> From 1700 to 1840, enslaved blacks were described as immune to mental illness. John Galt, M.D., medical director at Eastern Lunatic Asylum in Williamsburg, Va., hypothesized that enslaved Africans were immune from the risk of mental illness because they did not own property, engage in commerce, or participate in such civic affairs as voting or holding public office. The immunity hypothesis assumed that the risk of "lunacy" would be high est in those populations who were emotionally exposed to the stresses of profit making—principally wealthy white men.

Of course, this immunity hypothesis was later replaced by the Exaggerated Risk Hypothesis towards 1860, which predicted excess mental illness, dependency, and dangerousness of black people if slavery were abolished. Again, these observations link distress to the framework of politics and economics rather than health and wellbeing.

In the same way, we have observed that in Western Europe and America during the Cold War (1947–1991), the refugees that were escaping communist countries were treated as heroes. There was minimal discussion of trauma, PTSD, or distress among those refugees. Most of the refugees that were coming to capitalist countries were educated, and from similar cultural backgrounds, and the numbers were not high. However, the end of the Cold War experienced a surge of internal wars in Africa, Asia, Latin/South America, and the West Asia (Middle East). Suddenly, higher numbers of people from different cultural backgrounds were coming to Europe and North America. As Ingleby (2005) observed, since the end of the Cold War, there has been a parallel surge in research and articles related to mental health (or rather mental disabilities) of refugees. We wonder whether this too might be explained mostly by the political, economic, and social impacts of the refugee influx rather than a concern for the refugees' mental health and wellbeing. This close association of biomedicine, psychiatry and political and economic contexts is developed further in Chap. 3.

2.6 Global Concerns of Distress

This chapter has shown that mental health and wellbeing has become a commodity in the marketplace, which includes biomedical knowledge and biomedical practice. It is important to understand the MGMH, international and national NGOs, mental health educators and services, from this backdrop. Although there is a growing debate within the global mental health discourse regarding cultural concepts and traditional approaches, the underlying philosophy remains to locate distress in the individual and summon responses from the Euro-North American canon of interventions, whether pharmaceutical or talking therapies. Here, the mental health 'treatment gap' takes on epidemiological and ethical justifications to reduce suffering, and yet does so based on the rationale that by 'no treatment' means no biomedical treatment, ignoring its own literature reviews and research evidence on the role of traditional healing or other spiritual practitioners (Pham et al., 2021). Instead, Moitra et al. (2023) argue that all different kinds of distress are combined into mental illnesses or disorders. They point out that mental illness disproportionately affects vulnerable communities and argue that recent global events including geo-political events, environmental change, and the COVID-19 pandemic have all impacted mental health requiring coordinated psychosocial care and support for people that are in need (Moitra et al., 2023).

As we discussed earlier in this chapter, this raises the question of who decides the "need" for psychosocial care and support. Is that the affected population themselves or biomedical experts? This is the power imbalance we bring into the discussion in this book. Over the years, the development experts have increasingly discussed the importance of mental health, especially from a therapeutic and clinical perspective. Lengfelder (2017) in her Human Development Dialogue post argued that societies must fully integrate psychological therapies (assuming that they are biomedical interventions) into general health systems to make treatments accessible to everyone. What is missing here is who determines the character and focus of therapies or treatment. Even within the United Nations Development Programme, where the global push is to facilitate the expansion of capabilities and freedoms so that everyone can reach their potential, the discussion of mental health treatments is promoted within the same global or local contexts of social, political, cultural, economic, and environmental inequalities, exclusions, and discriminations that push people into distress. There is no discussion in current education, social, health and welfare institutions about facilitating people's internal capabilities and freedoms, or where people can better deal with the external challenges they face. In the same tone Lengfelder (2017) goes on to point out that while people in the USA and Germany are suffering from mental distress or illnesses, these two countries are described as "developed" and have "favourable external" conditions. And yet in the USA, 37.2 million people live in poverty (US Census Bureau, 2022), and in Germany 20.9% of the population are affected by severe deprivation (Statistisches Bundesamt, 2024). In 2017, CNN Business reported that in Germany, the richest 10% of the population owns 60% of assets, while the bottom 40% have almost nothing. According to the nonpartisan Congressional Budget Office (2021), the income inequalities in the USA has been steadily rising for many years. Without even pointing towards racial and class inequalities in these two countries, it is hard to understand what "favourable external" conditions Lengfelder is signalling. The point here is that 'development' as we understand it in the mainstream discourse has not enabled individuals to better deal with their external surroundings.

Lengfelder is not alone in this push towards the inclusion of mental health in development. In 2015, Izutsu et al. asserted that depression is a leading cause of disability worldwide. They argued that international actors had not mobilised the required efforts and resources to deal with such disability because the economic costs of mental disorders were so high. A decade on from the 2007 Lancet Series on global mental health, which pushed for a bio-medicalisation of mental health in policymaking, the Lancet Commission on global mental health and sustainable development started to push for the Sustainable Development Goals to include future directions for mental health (Patel et al., 2018). What this Commission proposed was for the global mental health agenda to be expanded to improve mental health of whole populations by reducing the 'treatment gaps' for mental disorders and to reduce the global burden of mental disorders by addressing prevention.

Yet at the same time the Global Risk Report by the World Economic Forum (2024) presented that the global outlook of the shocks generated by COVID-19, various conflicts and wars, and disasters will bring further shocks in world systems. For example, environmental risks through the climate crisis would create severe disruptions to the lives of billions of people across the world. Instead of dealing with these global risks through socio-cultural and political, systems, the MGMH is pushing for biomedical interventions as solutions to distress. A coloniality in the use of terms like mental disorders and mental illnesses, where collections of syndromes and symptoms are classified by psychiatrists and mental health experts in Euro-North American countries, is shown by the assumption that distress in Sri Lanka or Malawi can be seen in exactly the same way as in the Global North. What is being ignored is that mental disorders, mental illnesses, and even mental health itself occupy different meanings in different socio-cultural settings. The universalism in the MGMH is reproducing a colonial project. The colonised are spoken for and are unable to represent themselves—whether they are in Malawi or Sri Lanka. Instead, the MGMH explicitly claims to be a progressive movement, attempting to educate, improve, and reform populations everywhere, with Euro-North American knowledge as definitive. We conclude this chapter by asking questions that logically derive from such assertions and which this book will seek to address: who has the power to define a problem in any particular context, and whose knowledge is being called upon to solve that problem?

References

Allen, L. N., & Feigl, A. B. (2017). Reframing non-communicable diseases as socially transmitted conditions. *Lancet Global Health, 5*(7), e644–e646.

American Psychiatric Association. (2013). *Diagnostic and statistical manual of mental disorders: DSM-5* (5th ed.). American Psychiatric Publishing.

Argenti-Pillen, A. (2003). *Masking terror: How women contain violence in southern Sri Lanka*. University of Pennsylvania Press.

Bentall, R. P. (2010). *Doctoring the mind. Why psychiatric treatments fail*. Penguin Books.

Brossard, B., & Chandler, A. (2022). *Explaining mental illness; sociological perspectives*. Bristol University Press.

Bureau, US Census. (2022). *National poverty in America awareness month: January 2022*. https://www.census.gov/newsroom/stories/poverty-awareness-month.html

Carrozza, C. (2015). Democratizing expertise and environmental governance: Different approaches to the politics of science and their relevance for policy analysis. *Journal of Environmental Policy & Planning, 17*(1), 108–126.

Clark, J. (2014). Medicalization of global health 2: The medicalization of global mental health. *Global Health Action, 7*, 1.

CNN Business. (2017). *Rich Germany has an inequality problem. These numbers prove it.* https://money.cnn.com/2017/09/20/news/economy/germany-election-inequality-income/index.html#:~:text=The%20richest%2010%25%20the%20population%20owns%2060%25%20of,unemployment%20dropping%20to%20record%20lows%2C%20according%20to%20Grabka

Cohen, A., Padmavati, R., Hibben, M., et al. (2016). Concepts of madness in diverse settings: A qualitative study from the INTREPID project. *BMC Psychiatry, 16*, 388.

Cohen, B. M. Z. (2016). *Psychiatric hegemony; a Marxist theory of mental illness.* Palgrave Macmillan.

Congressional Budget Office. (2021). *The distribution of household income 2018.* https://www.cbo.gov/system/files/2021-08/57061-Distribution-Household-Income.pdf

Conrad, P., & Bergey, M. (2015). Medicalization: Sociological and anthropological perspectives. In J. D. Wright (Ed.), *International encyclopedia of the Social & Behavioral Sciences* (2nd ed., pp. 105–109). Elsevier Ltd..

Davis, K. (2018). Blacks are immune from mental illness. *Psychiatric News, 53*(9). https://psychnews.psychiatryonline.org/doi/full/10.1176/appi.pn.2018.5a18

Del Casino, V. J. (2004). (re)placing health and health care: Mapping the competing discourses and practices of 'traditional' and 'modern' Thai medicine. *Health & Place, 10*(1), 59–73.

European Commission. (2013). Flash Eurobarometer 338 – *Monitoring the social impact of the crisis: Public perceptions in the European Union* (WAVE 6), GESIS Data Archive: Cologne. 2013 Report No.:ZA5773.

Fernando, S. (2014). *Mental health worldwide: Culture, globalization, and development.* Palgrave Macmillan.

Frasquilho, D., Matos, M. G., Salonna, F., Guerreiro, D., Storti, C. C., Gaspar, T., & Caldas-de-Almeida, J. M. (2015). Mental health outcomes in times of economic recession: A systematic literature review. *BMC Public Health, 16*(1), 1–40.

Funtowicz, S. O., & Ravetz, J. R. (1993). Science for the post-normal age. *Futures, 25*(7), 739–755.

Helman, C. G. (2007). Cross cultural psychiatry. In C. G. Helman (Ed.), *Culture, health, and illness* (5th ed.). Hodder Arnold.

Henning, D. H. (2002). *A Manual for Buddhism and deep ecology* (Special Ed.). The World Buddhist University.

Holmes, T. H., & Rahe, R. H. (1967). The social readjustment rating scale. *Journal of Psychosomatic Research, 11*(2), 213–218.
Horwitz, A. V. (2003). *Creating mental illness.* University of Chicago Press.
Ingleby, D. (2005). *Forced migration and mental health: Rethinking the Care of Refugees and Displaced Persons.* Springer.
Izutsu, T., Tsutsumi, A., Minas, H., Thornicroft, G., Patel, V., & Ito, A. (2015). Mental health and wellbeing in the sustainable development goals. *The Lancet Psychiatry, 2*(12), 1052–1054.
Jackson, M. (2013). *The age of stress: Science and the search for stability.* Oxford University Press.
Jayawickrama, J. (2008). *Why is there more laughter in refugee camps than on the streets of London?* Royal Geographical Society / Institute of British Geographers.
Johnson, A. L. (2021). Changes in mental health and treatment, 1997–2017. *Journal of Health and Social Behavior, 62*(1), 53–68.
Jumbe, S., Nyali, J., Simbeye, M., Zakeyu, N., Motshewa, G., & Pulapa, S. R. (2022). 'We do not talk about it': Engaging youth in Malawi to inform adaptation of a mental health literacy intervention. *PLoS One, 17*(3), e0265530.
Kirmayer, L. J. (2012). Cultural competence and evidence-based practice in mental health; epistemic communities and the politics of pluralism. *Social Science and Medicine, 75*, 249–256.
Kleinman, A. (1977). Depression, somatization, and the new cross-cultural psychiatry. *Social Science and Medicine, 11*, 3–10.
Kleinman, A. (1980). *Patients and healers in the context of culture: An exploration of the borderland between anthropology, medicine, and psychiatry.* University of California Press.
Kleinman, A. (2006). *What really matters: Living a moral life amidst uncertainty and danger.* Oxford University Press.
Kleinman, A., & Good, B. (Eds.). (1985). *Culture and depression.* University of California Press.
Knipe, D. W., Gunnell, D., Pieris, R., Priyadarshana, C., Weerasinghe, M., Pearson, M., Jayamanne, S., Hawton, K., Konradsen, F., Eddleston, M., & Metcalfe, C. (2019). Socioeconomic position and suicidal behaviour in rural Sri Lanka: A prospective cohort study of 168,000+ people. *Social Psychiatry and Psychiatric Epidemiology, 54*, 843–855.
Kohn, R., Saxena, S., Levav, I., & Saraceno, B. (2004). The treatment gap in mental health care. *Bulletin of World Health Organisation, 82*(11), 858–866.
Lengfelder, C. (2017). *Mental health: A fundamental component of human development.* Human Development Reports. https://hdr.undp.org/content/mental-health-fundamental-component-human-development
Leventhal, H. O. R., & Ian, B. (2012). *The self-regulation of health and illness behaviour.* Routledge.

Littlewood, R., & Lipsedge, M. (1997). *Aliens and alienists: Ethnic minorities and psychiatry* (3rd ed.). Routledge.

Lund, C., Tomlinson, M., & Patel, V. (2015). Integration of mental health into primary care in low-income and middle-income countries: The PRIME mental healthcare plans. *British Journal of Psychiatry*, s1–s3.

McCracken, J. (2012). *A history of Malawi, 1859–1966*. Boydell & Brewer Ltd.

Mental Health Foundation. (2023). *Stress, anxiety and hopelessness over personal finances widespread across UK – New mental health survey*. https://www.mentalhealth.org.uk/about-us/news/stress-anxiety-and-hopelessness-over-personal-finances-widespread-across-uk-new-mental-health-survey

Mills, C. (2014). *Decolonizing global mental health: The psychiatrization of the majority world*. Routledge.

Mills, C., & Fernando, S. (2014). Globalising mental health or pathologising the global south? Mapping the ethics, theory and practice of global mental health. *Disability and the Global South, 1*(2), 188–202.

Moitra, M., Owens, S., Hailemariam, M., Wilson, K. S., Mensa-Kwao, A., Gonese, G., Kamamia, C. K., White, B., Young, D. M., & Collins, P. Y. (2023). Global mental health: Where we are and where we are going. *Current Psychiatry Reports, 25*(7), 301–311.

Moncrieff, J. (2009). *The myth of the chemical cure. A critique of psychiatric drug treatment*. Palgrave Macmillan.

Pascal, B. (2008). *Human Happiness*. Penguin Books.

Patel, V., & Prince, M. (2010). Global mental health: A new Global Health field comes of age. *Journal of the American Medical Association, 303*(19), 1976–1977.

Patel, V., Saxena, S., Lund, C., Thornicroft, G., Baingana, F., Bolton, P., Chisholm, D., Collins, P. Y., Cooper, J. L., Eaton, J., & Herrman, H. (2018). The lancet commission on global mental health and sustainable development. *The Lancet, 392*(10157), 1553–1598.

Pham, T. V., Koirala, R., Wainberg, M. L., & Kohrt, B. A. (2021). Reassessing the mental health treatment gap: What happens if we include the impact of traditional healing on mental illness? *Community Mental Health Journal, 57*, 777–791.

Pilecki, B. C., Clegg, J. W., & McKay, D. (2011). The influence of corporate and political interests on models of illness in the evolution of the DSM. *European Psychiatry, 26*, 194–200.

Prophecy Market Insights. (2023). *Global mental health market*. https://www.globenewswire.com/en/news-release/2022/06/22/2467263/0/en/Global-Mental-Health-Market-is-estimated-to-be-US-527-44-billion-by-2030-with-a-CAGR-of-3-40-during-the-forecast-period-By-PMI.html

Rabkin, J. G., & Struening, E. L. (1976). Life events, stress, and illness. *Science, 194*, 1013–1020.

Radhakrishnan, S. (1950). *The Dhammapada: With introductory essays, Pali text, English translation and notes*. Oxford University Press.

Radhakrishnan, S. (1963). *Bhagavad Gita*. George Allen and Unwin Ltd.

Sartorius, N., Jablensky, A., Korten, A., Ernberg, G., Anker, M., Cooper, J., & Day, R. (1986). Early manifestations and first-contact incidence of schizophrenia in different cultures: A preliminary report on the initial evaluation phase of the WHO collaborative study on determinants of outcome of severe mental disorders. *Psychological Medicine, 16*(4), 909–928.

Saxena, S., Jané-Llopis, E., & Hosman, C. (2006). Prevention of mental and behavioural disorders: Implications for policy and practice. *World Psychiatry, 5*(1), 5–14.

Statistisches Bundesamt. (2024). *Income, living conditions, risk of poverty*. https://www.destatis.de/EN/Themes/Society-Environment/Income-Consumption-Living-Conditions/Living-Conditions-Risk-Poverty/_node.html

Steinforth, A. S. (2009). *Troubled minds: On the cultural construction of mental disorder and normality in southern Malawi*. Peter Lang.

Stevenson, A. (2010). *Cultural issues in psychology*. Routledge.

Summerfield, D. (2008). How scientifically valid is the knowledge base of global mental health? *British Medical Journal, 336*(7651), 992–994.

UMDS MSc in General Practice Teaching Group. (1999). 'You're depressed'; 'no I'm not': GPs' and patients' different models of depression. *The British Journal of General Practice, 49*(439), 123–124.

Votruba, N., & Thornicroft, G. (2016). Sustainable development goals and mental health: Learnings from the contribution of the fundamental SDG global initiative. *Global Mental Health, 3*, E26.

White, R. G., & Sashidharan, S. P. (2014). Towards a more nuanced global mental health. *British Journal of Psychiatry, 204*, 415–417.

World Economic Forum. (2024). *The global risk report 2024* (19th ed.). World Economic Forum.

World Health Organisation. (2013). *Mental health action plan*. WHO.

World Health Organisation. (2016). *mhGAP intervention guide for mental, neurological and substance use disorders in non-specialized health settings*. Version 2.0. WHO.

World Health Organisation. (2023). *What is stress?* https://www.who.int/news-room/questions-and-answers/item/stress

World Health Organization. (2022). *ICD-11: International classification of diseases* (11th revision). https://icd.who.int/WorldHealthOrganisationICD

Wright, J., & Maliwichi-Senganimalunje, L. (2020). Pluralism and practicality: Village health Workers' responses to contested meanings of mental illness in southern Malawi. *Anthropology & Medicine, 27*(1), 32–48.

Wright, J., Mazumdar, P., Barua, D., Lina, S., Bibi, H., Kanwal, A., Mujeeb, F., Naz, Q., Safi, R., Ul Haq, B., & Rana, R. Z. (2020). Integrating depression care within NCD provision in Bangladesh and Pakistan: A qualitative study. *International Journal of Mental Health Systems, 14*, 1–13.

CHAPTER 3

Coloniality of the Biomedical Model

3.1 Coloniality of Knowledge and Knowledge as Power

> [A]ny western medical institution more than a century old and which claims to stand for peace and justice has to confront a painful truth—that its success was built on the savage legacy of colonialism.
> Horton (2019, p. 996).

In the previous chapter we have begun to make links between the knowledge system of biomedicine and how these ideas and practices that emerged from Europe and North America have come to dominate understandings of health worldwide in a manner that parallels colonialism. This chapter will take a deeper look at how this colonising process emerged and continues to be experienced in localities of Malawi and Sri Lanka. However, before going into further details in this chapter, we will define certain terms that relate to colonial power relations, and which may be helpful in navigating this chapter.

Based on Ferro (1997), and Howe (2002), we define colonisation as a process of establishing a dominance over a targeted geographical location or communities for the purpose of control. The Stanford Encyclopaedia of Philosophy (2023) defines colonialism as a practice of domination, which involves the conquest of one people by another. Within this context, we

J. Jayawickrama, J. Wright, *Under the Gaze of Global Mental Health*, The Politics of Mental Health and Illness,
https://doi.org/10.1007/978-3-031-78258-9_3

describe coloniality as long-standing patterns of power that emerged from colonialism, but that define culture, labour, relationships, and knowledge production beyond the limits and existence of colonial administrations (Maldonado-Torres, 2007). Coloniality outlives colonialism and is preserved in books, the criteria for academic performance, cultural patterns, "common sense", self-image, aspirations of self, and other aspects of modern experience (Quijano, 2000). Both Maldonado-Torres (2007) and Quijano (2000) explain coloniality of power as a force that shapes knowledge and determines what it means to be a person and is wielded by colonisers to assign some people and groups to the zone of sub-humanity. It is important to understand that these definitions function differently in different contexts. For example, in Malawi, the impact of colonialism and coloniality functions as a form of oppression that is visible within the socio-cultural sphere. In Sri Lanka, this is much more subtle, and functions primarily within knowledge and language. Regardless of the functionality, the coloniality of power is visible in everyday lives in both Malawi and Sri Lanka.

Whereas the industrial revolution in Europe in the nineteenth century has often been seen as a triumph of Western or European intellect and technological expertise, it is hard to dispute that it was achieved by the prerequisite of slavery and exploitation of resources. Likewise, conflict around the world that secured this imperialism and has been justified as righteous and the triumph of enlightenment thinking—from the crusades of the eleventh to thirteenth centuries to the East India Company of the seventeenth to nineteenth centuries, from Afghanistan to the Americas—was the exercise of economic and political oppression on a global scale. Recent analysis has traced Western imperialism through eras of genocide, slavery, and colonialism to depict the contact and relations between people and with a sharpened critique on the post-colonial world of new imperialism (Andrews, 2021) as a way of contextualising current relations and globalising endeavours including the promotion of 'health'. Whilst such writing is heralding something of a new recognition of the responsibilities and influence of Europe's colonial past, accounts from the Global South have been cultivated by writers such as Walter Mignolo and Ponna Wignaraja for many decades. The author Ngugi wa Thiongo (1986) has no illusions about the devastating impact and potential that colonisation still has on the world.

> Imperialism is total: it has economic, political, military, cultural and psychological consequences for the people of the world today. It could even lead to holocaust.
>
> Ngugi wa Thiongo (1986, p. 2).

With a similar focus on the colonialising of the mind, the psychologist, Bulhan (2015) provides an account of the impact of colonialism on the psychology of Africa. Writing from Somaliland, Bulhan defines the systemic and organised violence against not only peoples but their ideas of self and of their thoughts through different stages of colonialism.

Classic colonialism commenced with populations in Africa and the Indian subcontinent becoming "populations captive in their own lands" (Bulhan, 2015 p. 243) serving the economic and political demands of the coloniser. Tea, coffee, cotton, and other cash crops replaced centuries of mixed agriculture across the Indian subcontinent and Africa, with huge profits for the colonisers, but economic precariousness and environmental fragility for the local populations. Exploitation of valuable minerals produced similarly unstable livelihoods and inhuman conditions from the goldfields of Tanganyika to the diamond mines of South Africa and copper mines of Northern Rhodesia (Rodney, 1972). Any public infrastructure works too were undertaken to benefit the colonising power, with all road and rail links directed to the transportation of materials to international markets (Andrews, 2021). Indeed, Rodney has no patience for any 'balance sheet' of empire where the departed coloniser is credited for leaving behind valuable infrastructural resources. Instead, Rodney points to the fact that throughout Africa's colonisation, medical, education and social services were withheld from local populations for self-interested (primarily economic) motivations.

> [N]one of the wealth of exploited Africans could be deployed for the assistance of their brothers outside the money economy.
>
> Rodney (1972, p. 249).

Disinterest in anything that did not produce immediate material gain for the coloniser is Illustrated by the fact that in Nigeria in the 1930s twelve hospitals were constructed for the 4000 whites, while for the 40 million blacks there were only 52 hospitals. The training of local African medical workers was equally piecemeal ahead of independence (Rodney, 1972).

So, while historically, the European invasion of the Americas first pursued material exploitation and cultural domination, and the transatlantic slave trade further sequestered the resources required for European economic and political control, within these enterprises a cultural and psychological colonisation of the mind took place for both colonisers and the colonised. Race became the justification for such exploitation and superiority of whites (Bulhan, 2015) and what it is to be human was viewed through the prism of racism and construction of the 'other' (Said, 1991). With this came the colonisation of knowledge, including changing indigenous beliefs and philosophies for Christianity, with an insistence on capitalism, and an exchange of kinship ties and communalism for individualised monetised relations (Rodney, 1972).

Even following independence from colonial rule in the 1950s–1970s, continuities of servitude mirrored those seen in the 'emancipation' from slavery to indentured labour in the USA in the 1800s (Andrews, 2021) where despite a rhetoric of freedom, the economic conditions prolonged enslavement. In fact, although there is some dispute as to the profitability of Caribbean sugar plantations in the nineteenth century, the idea that an economic rather than humanitarian justification can be offered for emancipation is not without its advocates (Williams, 1964; Ryden, 2009). With a similar eye on economic advantage, the post-Second World War consensuses of victors established the five permanent members of the United Nations and put in place institutions and frameworks such as the International Monetary Fund (IMF), and World Bank (WB) and Bretton Woods agreements, that ensured trade and development matched the needs of these powers. Indeed, it has been argued that, again like the emancipation of slavery in the US, European countries held out against granting independence to their colonies until the 1950s–1970s when both economic frameworks and local infrastructure were in place to service these continuities (Rodney, 1972; Andrews, 2021).

In this way, within former colonial countries, systems were created for the imitation of colonial power by local elites, already schooled (literally, at US and European boarding schools and universities) in the same laws and institutions. As Bulhan explains:

> [The] flawed colonial state turned into a neocolonial machine that not only oppressed the people, but also worked to the advantage of former colonial powers and their allies.
>
> Bulhan (2015, p. 243).

All attempts by the emerging nations to carve a new 'non-aligned' direction were blocked by the old colonial powers' economic and politically sponsored violence, including assassinations (Tharoor, 2017). In such a light, the granting of independence appears fuelled less by the moral pursuit for dignity and human rights, and more that the global powers had established a new way of retaining economic and political influence through a 'neocolonialism'.

In the same way, the continuity of coloniality cemented the privilege of certain knowledge and values. For coloniality does not merely refer to the colonisation of indigenous culture in the Americas, but instead it refers to a whole system of thought, a mentality, and a power structure that constructs "the hegemonic and Euro-centred matrix of knowledge" (Mignolo, 2010, p. 11). 'Metacolonialism', as Bulhan (2015) terms it, extends benefits to the previous colonisers and the imperial power dynamics are retained. As a result, colonialism, and its successor coloniality, created the "racially hierarchised, imperialistic, colonialist, Euro-American-centric, Christian-centric, hetero-normative, patriarchal, violent and modern world order" (Ndlovu Gatsheni, 2013*)*, which cannot but infiltrate globalised thinking on what it means to be a person, to experience distress and to inform helping responses (Farley, 2003).

3.2 Psychiatry and the Exercise of Biomedical Power in the Colonies

Consistent with its dominance in all other sectors of society, the colonial powers established health and mental health services that aligned with the colonialist ideology and purpose at that time. Initially, for instance, western medicine in the colonies ignored the indigenous populations. Focus instead was on understanding and combatting the extreme mortality amongst European colonists across Africa, Asia and the Americas who were exposed to 'tropical' diseases. Indeed, the parallel mortality of indigenous populations was not only ignored but, in some cases, operationalised as a tool of oppression and at times extermination (Andrews, 2021). The health of locals began to take on relevance to colonialists once the economic costs of high morbidity and mortality and reduced productivity were seen to be threatening profit (Lyons, 1992). In fact, it was European exploration and early settlement from the fifteenth and sixteenth centuries onwards that prompted the growth of a tradition of discussion of what were called the diseases of warm or hot climates. On one level, tropical medicine was deeply involved in the political and social aspects of colonialism. Europeans, especially soldiers, public servants, and officials, had to move to the tropics, where the contraction of a life-threatening disease was a real danger. At the same time, indigenous people were subject to the same diseases, so the main source of labour used in European agriculture, such as sugar cane in the West Indies, was threatened (Farley, 2003). Thus, the reason for the existence of tropical medicine as a discipline was the protection of European colonial officials and the exploitation of indigenous workforce. The two schools of tropical medicine in the UK can therefore be seen to have a colonial foundation.

This ignorance of the indigenous person's health and situation was of course consistent with the overall consideration of the needs of the colonised and was justified within contemporary notions of racial superiority and its 'civilising mission' (Watt & Mann, 2011). Indeed, colonialism took the hegemony of a difference between 'higher' and 'lower' levels of 'civilisation' and stratified their systems accordingly. Where the biological sciences and emerging germ theory was interested in similarities of humans to explain vulnerability, exposure and immunity from communicable disease, the psychological and psychiatric theories focused on establishing 'difference'.

Not only in biomedicine, but also in the social sciences field, there was a European understanding of the differences between various races. In an Orwellian sense, they believed that some humans were deemed more equal than others. The European Enlightenment of the seventeenth and eighteenth centuries projected a notion of universal humanity, in which reason could be harnessed for the betterment of all humankind. However, this was concomitant with an interest in categorising "race" as a means of comprehending differences among humans. This parallel development emerged alongside the requirement to exploit raw materials, wherein colonisation necessitated the vilification of a 'savage' entity, depicted as morally and intellectually inferior to European culture and biology. Immanuel Kant (1764), for instance, posited that Africans inherently lacked emotions, stating that African natives naturally do not have feelings that are significant (Frierson & Guyer, 2012). Georg Wilhelm Friedrich Hegel (1770–1831) echoed similar sentiments, asserting that non-European "races" were inferior, lacking value, and devoid of progress potential. He also contended that "East Asians" were incapable of abstract thought (Andrews, 2021).

During what Bulhan (2015) framed as classical colonialism, psychologists and psychiatrists embarked on racial comparisons of the size of the brain, and from this concluded that Africans belonged to a lower evolutionary phase where mental disorders (from the European perspective) were non-existent. The absence of 'depression', for instance, was seen as directly attributed to a less evolved brain and contrasted the primitive 'noble savage' with a European's experience of self-blame and guilt as intimations of a civilised mind (Carothers, 1953). Such ideas of a less developed or childlike mind (Littlewood, 1996), advanced a notion of the vulnerability of people in the Global South to mental disorders that has resonance today; that of acculturation. Here psychiatrists in the nineteenth and early twentieth century saw the indigenous peoples as innately incapable of coping with 'modernity' which very lucidly implicates psychiatry in providing stereotypes that justified the colonial project.

> Certain races had particularly high rates of one sort of psychological illness or another through their position in the evolutionary chain and their ability (or failure) to dominate their nature. If melancholy was the fruit of European civilisation's gradual accumulation of culture and self-consciousness, then primitive mental illness – a lack of control over instinct and impulsivity – was demonstrated by tribal peoples.
>
> Madden, 1857, in Littlewood (1996, p. 247).

And yet psychiatry's essentialising of certain peoples and universalising of a biological psychiatry stood in contrast to some of the emerging social science literature where a number of scholars were shaping different understandings of the importance of culture to people's lives. Marcel Mauss in the 1920s showed the way that cultural expectation shaped emotional expectation (Mauss, 1926). Ruth Benedict uncovered different understandings of epilepsy in North America and in Siberia, concluding that concepts of normality and abnormality were socially allocated and reflecting of differing locally approved values and behavioural norms (Benedict, 1934) and, also in the 1930s, Margaret Mead provided evidence of cultural variation within other socialisation processes (Mead, 2001). Instead, in the face of this, psychiatry maintained the Kraepelin view that culture simply adds a context for what are essentially biological mental illnesses (Littlewood, 1996), which, despite its multiple limitations and critique (discussed in Chap. 2) still resonates with today's GMH movement.

However, it is reasonable to attest that psychiatry's ignoring of anthropological findings and cultural context was not universal and while much colonial psychiatry legitimised colonial rule as benign, 'rational', 'progressive', and just (Said, 1991), there were exceptions. Devereux (1939), for instance, devised a theory based on psychoanalysis that saw mental illness as resulting from an individual's disorientation and struggle with the complexities of a society. Other dissent from conventional psychiatric views emanated in the twentieth century from several schools of psychiatry located in the European colonies of North and East Africa. Here, variations in psychiatric discourse and practice were explored by trying to map the role and significance of 'culture' to the experience of psychological distress in Algiers (Keller, 2007), and in East Africa (Mahone, 2007), and there developed more socio-cultural understandings of mental illness, with some, such as in Senegal (Bullard, 2007) incorporating local aspects of healing. Also from North Africa, and albeit informed by European Freudian theory, Franz Fanon used his experiences as a psychiatrist during the Algerian War of Independence (1954–62) to highlight the profound psychological damage that resulted from the experience of being colonised. For Fanon, to be colonised was to be alienated from oneself and from one's environment, in just the same way as the person suffering from a psychiatric illness can be said to be alienated from his or herself (Fanon, 1952). This profound psychic damage, Fanon suggests, results in madness, and implicates the experience of being colonised and 'racialised' as fundamental to understanding personal and collective distress. Fanon's insights into the experience of both the oppressor and the oppressed carve out essential tenets of the colonial project that resonate still in contemporary attitudes to race and psychopathology.

However, at the time, colonial psychiatry in most countries across the Americas, Asia and Africa used medical and scientific 'credibility', to naturalise the colonisers as 'superior' while medicalising dissent and resistance to their rule (Mills, 2018, p. 210). In so doing Bulhan (2015, p. 246) suggests that such a process contested the very memory and reality of the colonised experience. As an example of psychiatry reflecting dominant values and mores of society, in 1851 Dr. Samuel Cartwright, a leading American pro-slavery psychiatrist, devised the psychiatric diagnosis of 'drapetomania' to pathologise slaves who attempted to escape captivity (Jackson, 2001). A century later, Carothers's (1953) characterisation of a 'kikuyu personality' was invoked to pathologise the resistance of Kenyans to colonial rule. Both represent ways in which psychiatry was implicated in the repression and violence of colonialism.

A question that arises from such determined scrutiny and policing of the colonised mind is of course the degree to which the institutions of colonial psychiatry can be seen as providing an instrument of social control in a form of what Foucault has termed *biopower* (Taylor, 2011) in the same way as psychiatry is critiqued in Europe. There are two aspects of this. On the one hand, the fact that psychiatry in the colonies did not take the form of a 'great confinement' of colonial populations in asylums (as there was in Europe and America) has led a number of scholars to be suspicious of the extent to which Foucault's idea of biopower could impact individual minds (e.g., Vaughan, 2007). However, if the spread of biomedicine is also seen as strongly attached to the practice of 'missionary medicine', which accompanied much colonial endeavour, then the reach of biomedicine outside of institutions becomes far more consuming. Greene and colleagues point out that whereby 'colonial medicine' focused on populations as 'collective' others (not individual self-conceptions), 'missionary medicine' was more interested in individuals (Greene et al., 2013 p. 47). More than simply treating illness, missionaries were converting individual souls to Christianity and, through notions of 'modernity', discrediting indigenous knowledge and values with a pernicious impact on the colonised. Megan Vaughan's work on mental health care in Malawi shows how the 'colonising mission' of psychiatry across the nineteenth and twentieth centuries was fuelled by racialist science and biology (Vaughan, 1991) in attempts to fortify the superiority of the colonisers. Such positions were used by colonial powers to exert political power and justify oppression through social control and human rights abuses (Mahone & Vaughan, 2007). Indeed, Mills (2014) has speculated from such historical comparisons that the current GMH movement is very much aligned to 'missionary medicine', and where 'biopower' becomes more palpable.

And after the colonial period, where one might have thought that independence of colonised countries would lead to differences in care and knowledge, most independent African countries continued to blindly follow the western 'science' of psychiatry (including retaining its mental health acts—Ibrahim, 2014). Following independence in 1947, India further advanced mental health care along Western lines, initially extending institutional care, followed by the extension of psychotherapeutic and drug treatments, and eventually moving from hospital to community care

(Wig, 2015). Malawi too followed on the acts left from British protectorate rule. Even the transcultural psychiatry movement that emerged in the 1950s and its search for cultural equivalents for "Western" emotional states can be seen as inextricably linked to the expansion of Western social systems (including medicine and psychiatry) through colonialism (Littlewood & Lipsedge, 1997). For Littlewood, and as we have seen in Chap. 2, 'pathology' carries with it a particular set of assumptions about normality and abnormality and "ignore(s) considerations of power and of the context of observation" (Littlewood, 1996, p. 259).

This domination and resultant cultural deprivation and epistemic injustice represent perhaps the most egregious and pervasive assault on the lives of the colonised. For, as with imperial notions that European explorers "discovered" new lands, these environments were home to peoples and societies, containing rich and sophisticated social, political, cultural, economic, and environmental contexts. Emboldened with ideas of western superiority and perception of threat, the colonisers response was an often-brutal intolerance of local, indigenous structures and thinking—even in aspects of health care. Ibrahim (2014) reports how the Kenyan colonial authority restricted and outlawed African healing systems and threatened healers with arrest and punishment as a way of colonising and depriving Africans of sacred and important cultural healing and educational systems (p. 396). Such sanctions had the effect of "displacing" communities from access to their own heritage and knowledge systems and began a process that continues today where non-biomedical approaches retreat into the extremities of societies (often rural village localities) mirroring the colonial era (Vaughan, 1991). So, what kind of indigenous philosophical thinking and traditional healing approaches in each of Malawi and Sri Lanka are being obscured by the advance of western medicine and what are the implications for local people?

3.3 The Coloniality of Mental Health in Malawi

Pre-colonial history in Malawi traces a common African heritage of early hunter-gatherer communities from 8000 BCE, and the emergence of pastoralists and farmers from 1300–1600 centuries CE. The 'Maravi' that settled in what is now Malawi share similarities in their historical, linguistic, and cultural practices deriving from migrations of Mang'anja, Chewa, Nyanja, Lomwe, and Yao peoples, in the thirteenth to sixteenth centuries and later the Ngoni peoples in the nineteenth century (Lwanda, 2005).

Shared appreciation of the significance of the environment, and particularly land ownership, provided the basis for significant social, political, religious, and cosmological ideas that shaped the cultures that developed. Advances in agricultural practices emerged and communities developed sophisticated systems of authority, governance, and thought that reflected a dependence on nature—with rituals of harvesting, planting, births, puberty, death, and prayers for rain all resonating within these traditional African cultures (Lwanda, 2008). A traditional comprehensive framework of health care and traditional healer practices also developed, shaped by the same cosmological and nature-based origins, and used to combat both individual illness and public health challenges such as epidemics and famine (Steinforth, 2009; Lwanda, 2008).

In colonial times the territory known as Malawi was ruled by the British as part of the British Central African Protectorate (1891 to 1907) and then up to 1953 as the British Protectorate of Nyasaland. The term protectorate refers to the determination of the British to 'protect' the region from Arab and Swahili slave traders in the north and Portuguese settlers in the south. From 1953 to 1963 the country continued to be governed by the British alongside the other British settler colonisers in Northern and Southern Rhodesia as the Federation of Rhodesia and Nyasaland until its independence in 1964.

As has been described earlier, while the primary motivation of colonisers is economic, the act of settlement brings with it exposure of the colonised (more vicariously than directly) to Western biomedicine. Indeed, the character of prominent nineteenth-century British explorers in East Africa, such as Dr. David Livingstone, Dr. John Kirk and Dr. Charles Mellor, link explorer, missionary, and medical movements (King & King, 1992), and this heralded over a century of at first British, and then wider international interest in the health of Malawians. The considerable influence of Scottish missionaries sought to establish a demonstrable link between education and health and led to a number of district hospitals, dispensaries and health centres being built across Malawi during the colonial period. These were all managed by white doctors and mainly serving white settler populations, military personnel, and administrative staff. However, post-independence saw the Malawian government investing more extensively in health services for its population, particularly supported in this by the missionary health services of the Christian Health Association of Malawi (CHAM), which supplemented the government provision of medical, maternity, and public health services and provided greater reach towards previously underserved rural populations. However, within the global context of post-1970s financial and economic governance, scarcity of resources has been a constant in the emergence of Malawi's health care provision, and the capacity to provide universal access to essential services has remained a relentless challenge. Messac (2020) has traced a continuity of official neglect of health care from colonial times, through the rule of first President Banda, and to subsequent national governments, who have all mobilised political, rhetorical, and martial campaigns to justify these scarcities in the face of such challenges. In terms of mental health care, the Zomba Lunatic Asylum in the southern region of Malawi was one of the earliest such institutions established in colonial Africa in 1910. For the period up until 1951 and its incorporation into the government medical department, the hospital was part of the Central Prison estate and was the only psychiatric facility in the country. Such an arrangement displays perhaps the main purpose of such an institution—to differentiate the 'mad' prisoners—and the stark conditions for in-patients mirrored that of prisoners. Historian Megan Vaughan has traced the emergence and significance of Zomba Mental Hospital within the context of colonial psychiatry and, in particular, how the Western biomedical underpinnings have reflected the development of European psychiatric thought (Vaughan, 1983)—moving through racialised theory and pathologising of the African mind, to confinement and incarceration, electro-convulsive therapy and drug treatments. Interestingly, writing in 1983, Vaughan writes:

> Today patients at Zomba Mental Hospital who express a wish to consult traditional healers in their homes are encouraged to do so. Alongside this increasing awareness of the value of traditional therapies, however, went the continued expansion of drug treatment, which is attested to by the massive increase in out-patients treated in the 1950s and the much more rapid turnover amongst in-patients.
>
> Vaughan (1983, p. 225).

Such a suggestion reminds us that the so-called development of thought—of, for instance, collaboration between biomedical and Traditional medicine systems—is by no means linear or progressive. Subsequent evidence from Zomba Mental Hospital and two other in-patient psychiatric facilities in the country (in the Northern and Central Regions) together with the rudimentary community mental health service provision, suggests a far less respectful relationship between the two systems (Steinforth, 2009; Wright & Maliwichi-Senganimalunje, 2020). To the Malawian throughout this time, the benefits of the Western health system of medicine (*mankhwala achizungu*—or 'white man's medicine') will have seemed far from obvious. Lwanda (2008) suggests that "western medicine appeared to have the same characteristics as traditional medicine: the rituals of history taking, diagnosis and treatment, but lacked the psycho-social and religious depth of traditional medicine" (p. 49). When it comes to mental health particularly, what it is to be a person (personhood) and to function ably in society, are all essential contextual sociocultural understandings. Traditional forms of medicine bear a direct connection to "traditional religious notions as well as other cultural concepts referring to Malawian cosmology" (Steinforth, 2009, p. 67). As we have seen, these Traditional African Religions have a commonality across sub-Saharan Africa and represent the major foundational philosophy—articulated either as distinct adherents to the religious and cultural tenets or, in the face of recurring waves of mission and evangelism, they are absorbed under the surface of proclaimed Islam and Christianity (Steinforth, 2009) in iconography, written and oral language (Ott, 2000), and characters represented in their beliefs, preaching, and healing practices—particularly the Christian Pentecostalist tradition (Strohbelm, 2005). As Schoffeleers (2000) says in his authoritative study of spirit beliefs and rituals in Malawi, "Traditional religion is still an important reality besides and within Christianity" (p. 7). So, within Malawi, and in different ethnic groups across the vast continent of Africa, with over centuries of invocation outside of and within organised religions, it is possible to distinguish core elements of a consistent Traditional African philosophy. As Acquah (2011) has suggested in his analysis of interactions between organised and traditional belief in Ghana,

> Indigenous religious beliefs and cultural values have served not only as the mediation of expressions for both indigenous Christians and Muslims … they have … shaped, to a great extent, the forms of Christianity and Islam that developed as well as the relationships between members of the diverse religious groups.
>
> Acquah (2011, p. 3).

Accordingly, Traditional African Religion forms the basis of the cultural life of most Africans (Acquah, 2020). Its central concept, *Ubuntu* (or in Malawi, *Umunthu*) can be described as both a normative philosophy and a value system that informs every aspect of living and promotes the wellbeing and personhood of individuals and the community. To possess an *umunthu* nature is to have learned particular attributes that shape an adult, with ethical reasoning and collective values. A person who possesses *umunthu* attitude is capable of compassion, reciprocity, mutuality and caring for their fellow human beings without discrimination (Goduka, 2000). Such notions position the person both within the larger cosmological context of the human life cycle (Steinforth, 2009) and within their community. Key to each is the respectful observance of certain *miyambo*—social mores/rules of living / personal characteristics to ways of behaving which are embedded in traditional cosmology and underpin notions of *umunthu* personhood.

Three key elements help explain central values of being a person.

1. Interconnectedness: *Umunthu* as a philosophy can only be operationalised through relationships. The expression, *I am because we are*, is the best example of this aspect. This points towards an understanding that an individual's sense of being cannot be separated from the family, community, and social context. This interconnectedness also surpasses time and place in that each person is themselves understood in context of relations with people/generations now deceased, so people have a connectedness with ancestors and on to higher being (God). The central importance of ancestors in their lives is indicated by the belief that ancestors are responsible for protecting and supporting their living relatives (Crawford & Maurice Lipsedge, 2004). Such a perspective influences an individual's subjective and emotional response to human experiences of disasters, conflicts, and uneven development.
2. Inclusion: As a collective philosophy and operational methodology, *Umunthu* promotes the oneness with everyone and everything around the individual. In this realisation, compassion, care, respect, and dignity are shared values. *Umunthu* advocates the moral value of the importance of collaboration in the face of crisis. It is important to understand that in a region where populations have experienced colonial looting, social, political, economic, cultural and environmental disorder, the collective action and mutual assistance have been essential for survival.
3. Inter-relationships: *Umunthu* provides a pragmatic framework for the relationship between the individual and the collective. Within

this framework, there is no space for dissecting life into fragmented pieces but to realise life in inclusion. This realisation of inclusion does not facilitate an understanding of mental health as a separate concept, but as an integral part of wellbeing of the individual that exists within the collective. *Umunthu* does not have the Cartesian divide of body and soul—or by the same virtue, dividing mental from physical—but rather represents a "complex spiritual-somatic unity" (Morris, 1994, p144). In this way, when external/structural factors/threats to people, and the assault on traditional *umunthu* values and *miyambo* are implicated as causality of distress, these social aspects are accommodated in the formulation of the distress—and action sought in their resolution. Living communally and holding as vital particular ways that a person should behave in his or her personification of *Umunthu* is a significant factor that differentiates perceptions of effective treatment from much Western and biomedical approaches where the individual is treated. Traditional healers treat the whole person, family, and community in a collective healing process. Indeed since 'formulations' also include understanding and identifying the source of the problem, a person is not considered treated until having undertaken traditional rituals that satisfy social requisites (Kirmayer, 2004; Steinforth, 2009).

These key traditional underpinnings that resonate understandings of mental health and wellbeing are surely vital to an understanding of and resolution to a person's distress. There is an abundance of wisdom and experience within such tenets that can be levelled at a person's experience of distress. And yet such notions fail to feature in MGMH interventions, which instead seek to identify and diagnose, and to deliver Western evidenced (usually pharmacological) interventions. As Farley (2003) puts it, through imperial policies and attitudes, Western medical practitioners define the type of medical system to be imposed on the indigenous population; they dictate which diseases are important and worthy of study, which diseases are to be controlled, and which control methods are to be used. In Malawi, therefore, both internally through the dominant biomedical system and from the backing of Western donors, it is the biomedical establishment that is consulted over the way forward for health problems, with all the limitations of cultural difference and preference, with no regard for indigenous knowledge and experience.

In the same way, when the call was raised in 2010 to establish a task-shifting educational initiative to build the capacity of community mental health care in Malawi, the project focus was on implementation—design, delivery, and evaluation—with no time for examining the existing environment and community perceptions. Indeed, why bother to explore further when common mental disorders, and a few psychotic disorders, were expected in the populations and the need was to identify cases, diagnose and treat with certain (Western) evidenced interventions? Given such a scenario, with the exercise of a powerful professional elite over the values and experience of ordinary people, it's very hard to distinguish this from colonialism. Indeed, the active engagement of both Malawian health professionals and external 'partners' and resources extend the equivalence more to the continuities of coloniality, where patterns of power and domination are accepted as convention (Maldonado-Torres, 2007) and there is an imitation of colonial power by local elites (Bulhan, 2015). In fact, the most striking reflection the second author (JW) noted from his earliest endeavours working with the Malawi health system, was the level of respect and deference afforded him in almost every encounter and the access to high officials in the health and government services by virtue of his position as a Western professional. This was in sharp contrast to his experience as a nurse in the UK where professional hierarchies ensured you seldom consulted anyone beyond your line manager, and certainly, no one was likely to consult you. But in Malawi his 'expertise' was not questioned, and he could see from his first days in the country how such prestige and access could become very seductive. Similar reflections on the impact of such outsider influence on the Malawian health professionals engaged in this mental health task-shifting project, including experiences of resistance, are discussed further in Chap. 4.

3.4 The Coloniality of Mental Health in Sri Lankan

Sri Lanka was colonised by the Portuguese, Dutch, and then the British from 1505 to 1948. This long period of colonialism destroyed the social, cultural, and political structures and evolution of the country, including the traditional medical systems. The foundations of the current Sri Lankan health care system were laid down in 1858 in the British colonial period. Florence Nightingale observed the efforts to establish a public health department in India by the British colonial government, and commented that it was indeed virtuous in effort, and a part of the mission to bring higher civilization to India (Cook, 1914). From the beginning Sri Lankan doctors trained in Western medicine, mainly from the UK, were providers of state medical care in hospitals and dispensaries. The Colombo medical school, founded in 1870, was crucial in the extension of the health care services as it was from these Colombo trained professionals that pressure for the extension of the health services to the general population came. The two decades of self-government before independence, following the Donoughmore Constitution in 1931 and the instigation of universal suffrage, contributed to a further rapid expansion of health services as politicians sought support from the electorate. The devastating 1934–1935 Malaria epidemic, with its estimated 80,000–100,000 deaths, was instrumental in extending the health infrastructure to previously neglected rural regions and exposed the widespread poverty of the Sinhala peasants who constituted most of the population. It also entrenched welfarism (free health care, food subsidies, and free education) in nationalist politics and shaped public policy and state interventionism in the first three decades after independence. Free education was also particularly salient for health; by the end of the colonial period, Sri Lanka was notable for its levels of female literacy—44% by the mid-1940s. Since women are deemed the principal health providers in Sri Lankan families and communities, this was a significant contributing factor to this health record.

The experience of the traditional medical systems—principally Ayurveda, alongside Siddha and Unani—was also singular in the colonial period. In the 1920s and 1930s the colonial government established and subsidised a Board of Indigenous Medicine, a training college, and a hospital. Although funded minimally compared with expenditure on biomedical services, traditional medicine was from the onset of independence an integral part of the official medical landscape. In addition, indigenous medicine in Sri Lanka places great value on good health and eschews any fatalistic attitude to illness, and such cultural norms fostered a health-seeking behaviour that encouraged accessing medical aid in whatever form. Hence, medical pluralism was firmly established.

By the 1920s, Sri Lanka had developed an extensive preventive health care system. In 1926 as a collaborative venture between the Rockefeller Foundation and the colonial government, a Health Unit was established at Kalutara. The programme of work of this first health unit included maternity and child welfare services, health education, sanitary work, communicable diseases work and school medical inspections. In 1937 malaria control work was also incorporated into health unit programmes concurrently with a multiplication of such units. The purpose of the health unit was preventive not curative and as they expanded across the island, they formed the basis of the primary health care infrastructure that continues to this day. According to the policy of Sri Lanka, the district is considered as the basic service unit and each district is under the direction of several Medical Officers of Health (MOH) depending on the size of the population, under which the policy is to establish Primary Community Mental Health Centers (PCMHC) in every district hospital in each MOH area.

Until the 1990s, the use of mental health services in Sri Lanka was limited to hospital care. In 1839 Governor Mackenzie introduced an ordinance to establish lunatic asylums. The mentally ill patients were housed in a leprosy asylum in Hendala (in the Western Province) during this period. A building of a separate asylum in Borella close to the city of Colombo was started in 1846 (Wambeek, 1866) and patients from Hendala Leprosy asylum were transferred to Borella in 1847. The new asylum provided protection and occupational therapy as the main mode of treatment, however, as a singular overcrowded institution, in practice many mentally ill people in Sri Lanka continued to be imprisoned in jails elsewhere on the island. The next new mental hospital was not built until nearly a century later in 1926 at Angoda in the Western Province and provided facilities for 1728 patients. The environment and treatment regime were no different from the previous asylum and, since it soon became overcrowded, no new treatment modalities were available.

A mental health policy drafted by the Sri Lanka College of Psychiatrists was approved by the Government of Sri Lanka for the first time in 2005 (Mental Health Policy, 2005). The objective of the policy was to decentralise the psychiatric services from the large mental hospitals in Colombo and to establish a community mental health service. A minimum of one acute psychiatric in-patient unit (APIU) based in each District General Hospital and a rehabilitation unit were planned to be established in each district. A community mental health team comprising of a Medical Officer of Mental Health (MOMH), Community Mental Health Nurses and a Community Support Officer was to be attached to each PCMHC. Medical officers who successfully complete the Diploma training programme were appointed as the Medical Officer of Mental Health in the community team.

In the Sri Lankan context, traditional knowledge and ways of thinking exist within traditional administrative systems, social systems, irrigation, legal practices, architecture, art, religious beliefs, and literature. According to Kusumaratne (2005), Sri Lankan indigenous medicine understands a healthy person as someone who has a balanced condition of bodily elements, digestion and metabolism, and stool extraction, with pleasant experiences of physical, social, and mental worlds. This definition of health includes the internal and external interconnectedness of the human being, which is not separated as a specialisation of mental health. To understand the mental health and wellbeing within the Sri Lankan context, therefore, it is important to understand the existing practices within communities. Much of this account is based on the first author's experiences of growing-up and living in Sri Lanka within different communities across the country. Many of the rituals and practices related to mental health and wellbeing are based on Buddhist, Hindu, and traditional philosophical understandings of life, living, and challenges. Chanting *Pirith* (Buddhist sutras) or *Mantras* (Hindu texts), *Bodhi Poojas* (offerings to the tree of Bodhi), meditation, astrology, healing through spirits, *Tovil* (psychodramas), charms and amulets, are common practices that can be seen in contemporary rural Sri Lanka.

Chanting *Pirith* or *Mantras* of the Buddhist or Hindu texts to overcome the challenges of life, fear, sadness, and requesting for protection from the Tripe Gem, (Buddha, Dharma, and Snagha) or divine entities is a common practice, which can be seen as an individual or group ritual. The practice of *Bodhi Pooja* is to present various offerings to the Bodhi tree, which is believed to be the tree under which the Prince Siddhartha meditated to become the Buddha. Bodhi Pooja ritual includes bathing the tree with water, offering flowers, hanging flower garlands, or flags on the tree. In doing this, the individual or group expect strength and courage to deal with the suffering they are facing through life.

Meditation has been a practice in which the person trains their mind to effectively deal with physical, mental, emotional, and spiritual challenges. Various meditation practices can be seen in Hindu and Buddhist communities mainly. However, the Christian and Catholic as well as Islamic prayers has various meditative elements, which provides the same benefits. Meditation practices in Sri Lanka can be divided into two different domains. One is through meditation classes conducted by various practitioners. This includes Buddhist monasteries that offer retreats, as well as different religious practices. This is very much dominated by Buddhist and Hindu religious practices. Second is personal meditation practices based on daily religious rituals. These are visible mostly in Buddhist and Hindu practices, however, different Christian/Catholic sects, and Islamic sects are practising different types of meditation without a label.

Astrology or Jyotishya (science of light) is a common practice within Buddhist and Hindu communities, which seeks to predict the future of an individual. It is most frequently evoked for naming a child, the first menstruation celebration, identifying a partner, marriage, starting a new business, and engaging in agriculture. However, when people are going through various social, physical, mental, or emotional challenges, it is also a common practice to seek advice from an astrologer, who will recommend various rituals to deal with challenges.

The traditional practice of *Tovil* (psychodramas) is less and less practised in Sri Lanka. This is mainly due to the lack of expert practitioners as well as the modern medicine claims that these psychodramas are useless in dealing with mental health and wellbeing. For example, a form of psychodrama, which deals with 18 ailments of blindness, paralysis, excess heat, body sores, insanity, dumbness, ear diseases, delirium, death, vomiting, diarrheal diseases, nausea, evil dreams, loss of consciousness, bile-related diseases, rheumatism, and epilepsy has been utilised by practitioners who are expert in addressing the 18 demons that are responsible for these ailments. This practice of psychodrama is undertaken in public, and involves drumming, music, chanting, and many other ritualistic practices. Together this combines a therapeutic encounter for the patient, an entertaining public gathering of friends and relatives, and a religious discourse.

Despite the continuance of each of these diverse healing traditions, albeit in fewer and more restricted forms and localities, the increasing dominance of the Western biomedical system has been uninterrupted. According to Goonatilake (1998), in the Sri Lankan context, through the many decades of coloniality, Western knowledge has become the acceptable worldview, and is studied in schools and universities. This very process of legitimising the Euro-North American knowledge in Sri Lanka (and South Asia) has had the effect of delegitimising traditional knowledges without critical examination or understanding of the cost.

3.5 The Mind in Social Life

Since the mind is undeniably embedded in social life, the standardisation and universalism of psychiatry that perpetuated throughout colonialism and on into postcolonial experiences of newly independent countries, may be seen as representing an assault on the pre-existing norms and values of the colonised.

Of course, what is being proposed here is a link between colonialism and biomedicine, and to many this may appear too simplistic and unnecessarily divisive. Certainly, European colonialism and biomedicine—as an articulation of post-enlightenment thinking and Western perceptions of modernity and 'public good'—are intimately linked. Some have very reasonably argued that in contrast to a colonial approach that benefitted only the few, the many biomedical advances in the control of communicable and non-communicable diseases have benefitted wider populations including the 'colonised' (Lock & Nguyen, 2010). And yet this surely demonstrates the same point. Whether of positive or negative benefit, the power of colonialism is held in its ability to privilege biomedicine and obscure or silence other knowledge systems. For the continued dominance of biomedicine within the formal health care sector, in the face of manifest pluralistic understandings within communities' informal care and traditional health care systems, is indicative of the colonial endeavour by representing the explicit hierarchy of Western over non-Western knowledge systems (Ibrahim, 2014; Fernando, 2014) and rendering powerless indigenous and collective understandings from Sri Lanka and Malawi.

In all these contexts, the appropriate way to frame distress is always through Western questions and categories. As Littlewood (1996, p. 259) offers,

> [I]t is not that psychiatry's inevitable grid, pathology, is necessarily inappropriate for comparing what looks to the European like 'suffering' or 'madness' in different societies, but pathology is just one possible grid and one which carries with it a particular set of assumptions about normality and abnormality which explicitly ignores consideration of power and of the context of observation. And of what it observes, and how 'observation' shapes it.

These two case examples from Malawi and Sri Lanka demonstrate the impact of power over peoples and their thinking. Not only this, in such a system, 'mental health' can be seen to be serving the function of

> the expansion of capitalism: it encourages consumption; it opens up new markets for products (most obviously in contemporary society, the markets for psychopharmaceuticals); it medicalizes resistance to capitalism; and, perhaps most importantly, it naturalizes and reproduces the norms and values of capitalism as common sense and take-for-granted conceptions of how the world should be.
>
> Cohen (2019, p. 32).

Bulhan (2015) sees colonialism as today more entrenched objectively and subjectively than it was in the past, and none could be more evident than in the operationalisation of GMH through its research and call for 'mental health literacy' and task-shifting educational interventions. The 'psychocentrism' dominant in such perspectives becomes an issue of social justice (Croft et al., 2016) and within such critiquing the pseudoscientific generalisability and universalism of psychiatry and psychiatrisation approaches of GMH, there are echoes of the 1920s Indonesian physicians' denounciation of 'psychiatric fascism' (Vaughan, 2007). Fanon (1952) and others certainly demonstrate psychiatry's witness to the violence of colonialism, and yet the extent to which Western psychiatry informs the hegemony of a society's beliefs, language and values has been disputed. Littlewood is less convinced that colonial psychiatry did this—since institutional psychiatry had very limited reach into the communities of the colonised—but he did concede that it does leave colonial residues in conceptualisations and expressions of mental illness (Littlewood, 1996). However, the activity of GMH, with its link to globalisation and its neoliberal agenda, represents a hegemony on another scale entirely, promoting a psychocentrism that threatens local indigenous knowledge and responses and social justice. The following chapter will extend this discussion by presenting how people experience, respond, and seek help for their distress, all under the gaze of GMH efforts.

References

Acquah, F. (2011). *The Impact of African Traditional Religious Beliefs and Cultural Values on Christian-Muslim Relations in Ghana from 1920 through the Present: A Case Study of Nkusukum-Ekumfi-Enyan area of the Central Region.* PhD Thesis, University of Exeter.

Acquah, F. (2020). Building bridges and trust through interfaith relations in Africa: The role of African indigenous religious and cultural values. *International Journal of African and Asian Studies, 66*, 32–44.

Andrews, K. (2021). *The new age of empire: How racism and colonialism still rule the world*. Penguin UK.
Benedict, R. (1934). Anthropology and the abnormal. *Journal of General Psychiatry, 10*, 59–80.
Bulhan, H. A. (2015). Stages of colonialism in Africa: From occupation of land to occupation of being. *Journal of Social and Political Psychology, 3*(1), 239–256.
Bullard, A. (2007). In S. Mahone & M. Vaughan (Eds.), *Imperial networks and postcolonial Independence: The transition from colonial to transcultural psychiatry*. Palgrave Macmillan.
Carothers, J. C. (1953). *The African mind in health and disease*. World Health Organisation.
Cohen, B. M. Z. (2019). A postcolonial critique of mental health: Empire and psychiatric expansionism. In R. Moodley & E. Lee (Eds.), *The Routledge international handbook of race, culture and mental health*. Routledge.
Cook, E. (1914). *The life of Florence nightingale* (Vol. 2). Macmillan and Company.
Crawford, T. A., & Maurice Lipsedge, M. (2004). Seeking help for psychological distress: The interface of Zulu traditional healing and Western biomedicine. *Mental Health, Religion & Culture, 7*(2), 131–148.
Croft, L., Gray, M., & Rimke, H. (2016). Mental health and distress as a social justice issue: Guest editors' preface and acknowledgments. *Studies in Social Justice, 10*, 1.
Devereux, G. (1939). A sociological theory of schizophrenia. *Psychoanalytic Review, 26*, 315–342.
Fanon, F. (1952). *Black skin, white masks*. Grove Press.
Farley, J. (2003). *Bilharzia: A history of Imperial tropical medicine*. Cambridge University Press.
Fernando, S. (2014). *Mental health worldwide: Culture, globalization and development*. Palgrave Macmillan.
Ferro, M. (1997). *Colonization*. Routledge.
Frierson, P., & Guyer, P. (Eds.). (2012). *Critical guide to Kant's observations on the feeling of the beautiful and the sublime*. Cambridge University Press.
Goduka, I. N. (2000). Indigenous/African philosophies: Legitimizing spirituality Centred wisdoms within academy. In P. Higgs, N. C. G. Vakalisa, T. V. Mda, & N. A. Assie-Lumumba (Eds.), *African voices in education*. Juta and, Ltd..
Goonatilake, S. (1998). *Toward a global science: Mining civilizational knowledge*. Indiana University Press.
Greene, J., Basilico, M. T., Kim, H., & Farmer, P. (2013). Colonial medicine and its legacies. In P. Farmer, J. Y. Kim, A. Kleinman, & M. Basilico (Eds.), *Reimagining global health: An introduction*. University of California Press.
Horton, R. (2019). Transcending the guilt of global health. *The Lancet, 394*(10203), 996.
Howe, S. (2002). *Empire: A very short introduction*. Oxford University Press.

Ibrahim, M. (2014). Mental health in Kenya: Not yet Uhuru. *Disability and the Global South, 1*(2), 393–400.

Jackson, V. (2001). *In our own voice: African-American stories of oppression, survival and recovery from mental health system.* [Online] In Our Own Voice: African American Stories of Oppression Survival And – DocsLib.

Keller, R. C. (2007). Taking science to the colonies: Psychiatric innovation in France and North Africa. In S. Mahone & M. Vaughan (Eds.), *Psychiatry and empire.* Palgrave Macmillan.

King, M. S., & King, E. (1992). *The story of medicine and disease in Malawi.* The Montefort Press.

Kirmayer, L. J. (2004). The cultural diversity of healing: Meaning, metaphor and mechanism. *British Medical Bulletin, 69*, 33–48.

Kusumaratne, K. L. S. (2005). *Indigenous medicine in Sri Lanka: A sociological analysis.* Sarasavi Publishers.

Littlewood, R. (1996). Psychiatry's culture. *International Journal of Social Psychiatry, 42*(4), 245–268.

Littlewood, R., & Lipsedge, M. (1997). *Aliens and alienists: Ethnic minorities and psychiatry* (3rd ed.). Routledge.

Lock, M., & Nguyen, V.-K. (2010). *An anthropology of biomedicine.* Wiley-Blackwell.

Lwanda, J. (2005). *Politics, culture and medicine in Malawi.* Kachere Series.

Lwanda, J. C. (2008). *Colour, class and culture: A preliminary communication into the creation of doctors in Malawi.* Duda Nsomba Publications.

Lyons, M. (1992). *The colonial disease: A social history of sleeping sickness in northern Zaire 1900–1940.* Cambridge University Press.

Mahone, S. (2007). East African psychiatry and the practical problems of empire. In S. Mahone & M. Vaughan (Eds.), *Psychiatry and empire.* Palgrave Macmillan.

Mahone, S., & Vaughan, M. (Eds.). (2007). *Psychiatry and empire.* Palgrave Macmillan.

Maldonado-Torres, N. (2007). On the coloniality of being: Contributions to the development of a concept. *Cultural Studies, 21*(2–3), 240–270.

Mauss, M. (1926). A definition of the collective suggestion of the idea of death. In *Sociology and psychology* (Mauss, Trans.). Routledge and Kegan Paul.

Mead, M., (2001). *Sex and temperament in three primitive societies* (1st Perennial ed.). Harper Collins.

Messac, L. (2020). *No more to spend: Neglect and the construction of scarcity in Malawi's history of health care* (Online ed.). Oxford Academic.

Mignolo, W. (2010). Introduction: Coloniality of power and de-colonial thinking. In W. Mignolo & A. Escobar (Eds.), *Globalization and the decolonial option* (pp. 1–21). Routledge.

Mills, C. (2014). *Decolonizing global mental health: The psychiatrization of the majority world*. Routledge.
Mills, C. (2018). The mad are like savages and the savages are mad: Psychopolitics and the coloniality of the psy. In B. M. Z. Cohen (Ed.), *Routledge international handbook of critical mental health*. Routledge.
Morris, B. (1994). *Anthropology of the self: The individual in cultural perspective*. Pluto Press.
Ndlovu Gatsheni, S. J. (2013). Why decoloniality in the 21st century. *The Thinker, 48*, 10.
Ngugi wa Thiongo. (1986). *Decolonising the mind: The politics of language in African literature*. James Currey.
Ott, M. (2000). *African theology in images*. CLAIM.
Quijano, A. (2000). Coloniality of power and eurocentrism in Latin America. *International Sociology, 15*(2), 215–232.
Rodney, W. (1972). *How Europe underdeveloped Africa*. Pambazuka Press.
Ryden, D. (2009). *West Indian slavery and British abolition, 1783–1807*. Cambridge University Press.
Said, E. W. (1991). *Orientalism: Western perceptions of the orient*. Penguin.
Schoffeleers, M. (2000). *Religion and the dramatisation of life: Spirit beliefs and rituals in southern and Central Malawi*. CLAIM.
Stanford Encyclopaedia of Philosophy. (2023). *Colonialism*. Stanford University Press.
Steinforth, A. S. (2009). *Troubled minds: On the cultural construction of mental disorder and normality in southern Malawi*. Peter Lang.
Strohbelm, U. (2005). *Pentecostalism in Malawi: A history of the apostolic faith Mission in Malawi*. Kachere.
Taylor, C. (2011). Biopower. In D. Taylor (red.), *Michel Foucault: Key concepts* (pp. 41–54). Acumen Publishing Ltd.
Tharoor, S. (2017). *Inglorious empire: What the British did to India*. Scribe Publications Pty Limited.
Vaughan, M. (1983). Idioms of madness: Zomba lunatic asylum, Nyasaland, in the colonial period. *Journal of Southern African Studies, 9*(2), 218–238.
Vaughan, M. (1991). *Curing their ills: Colonial power and African illness*. Polity Press.
Vaughan, M. (2007). Introduction. In S. Mahone & M. Vaughan (Eds.), *Psychiatry and empire*. Palgrave Macmillan.
Wambeek, J. (1866). *Report on lunatic asylum of Borella*. Colombo National Archives.
Watt, C. A., & Mann, M. (Eds.). (2011). *Civilizing missions in colonial and post-colonial South Asia: From improvement to development*. Anthem Press.

Wig, N. N. (2015). The beginnings of psychiatry in India. In S. Malhotra & S. Chakrabarti (Eds.), *Developments in psychiatry in India: Clinical, research and policy perspectives* (pp. 3–12). Springer.
Williams, E. E. (1964). *Capitalism & slavery*. A. Deutsch.
Wright, J., & Maliwichi-Senganimalunje, L. (2020). Pluralism and practicality: Village health Workers' responses to contested meanings of mental illness in southern Malawi. *Anthropology & Medicine, 27*(1), 32–48.

CHAPTER 4

Behind the 'Global Mental Health' Gaze

4.1 The Global Mental Health Gaze

> Biological beings become human beings through their engagement with the meanings and practices of their social world.
>
> Markus and Hamedani (2007, p. 32).

Markus and Hamedani's (2007) assertion give thought to how the social world frames people's experience and understanding of what it is to be human—including distress or mental health problems. These experiences are shaped from their social world and cannot be separated from their context. And yet this chapter provides examples of how one view of distress—the biomedical view—has assumed dominant status in global health efforts and with powerful institutions and professions dispensing this view as a universal experience and remedy. In response, this chapter will explore examples from Sri Lanka and Malawi that detail the lived experiences, impact and responses of people and health workers based on the research literature and the authors' experiences. Pluralistic health systems naturally possess different players and agendas, different weightings of power and differing expectations and responses. This chapter provides an analysis of the GMH agenda that harbours links with an imperial age, and whose detail offers that what might appear obvious often obscures reality and what is planned is often not what is delivered.

J. Jayawickrama, J. Wright, *Under the Gaze of Global Mental Health*, The Politics of Mental Health and Illness,
https://doi.org/10.1007/978-3-031-78258-9_4

In this chapter, we explain global mental health as a gaze. A solid intent that has colonised the minds of people in both Sri Lanka and Malawi. In our own conversations with elites in Malawi and Sri Lanka, there is a strong acceptance of global mental health categories of anxiety, depression, stress, and distress that needs "expert" help. In Lilongwe and Blantyre in Malawi as well as Colombo, Kandy, and Galle in Sri Lanka, the main cities, there are many individual counselling services that can be found easily. However, our focus is on people that are not part of the wealthy classes in Malawi or Sri Lanka. While people in Malawi and Sri Lanka are affected in similar ways through the gaze of GMH, we argue that among the poor and disadvantaged populations, this creates a double bind. The bind of poverty and bind of labels of mental health. In that, we are elaborating the mental health task-shifting project in Malawi (2010–2015) and the 2004 tsunami responses in Sri Lanka as two case examples. By no means do these two case studies provide a complete picture of Malawian or Sri Lankan mental health responses, but they do provide insights into the challenges and limitations of exerting 'outsider' knowledges on people's experiences of distress.

4.2 Understanding Mental Health in Malawi

Every joy will follow in grief's footsteps.
A Malawian proverb.

As we have seen in Chap. 3, 'task shifting' represents the major tool in the GMH armoury for responding to the problem of a treatment gap (with all assumptions contained within it) defined through the notion of the 'burden' of mental illness. Training cadres of staff in certain interventions seeks to increase access and coverage, and in particular attends to the problem of the lack of mental health care professionals required for the GMH project. From its emergence in 1990s in HIV/AIDS testing and rollout of antiretroviral medication (ARVs) and development in the 2000s primarily to fill capacity where human resource capacity was limited, there have been different types of task-shifting involving different cadres of health worker (Okoroafor & Christmals, 2023). In the case of mental health care in Malawi, this was one of the first adopters of the mental health task-shifting model. Undertaken in the Southern Region of Malawi 2010–15 the project sought to increase the availability of mental health support at community level by equipping the village-based health workers (or Health Surveillance Assistants (HSAs) as the health service termed them) to respond to the needs of people with mental health problems in the community. Populations in this essentially rural environment, with small trading centres and one large urban centre (Zomba), are primarily engaged in small-scale farming and trading and a subsistence economy. People's lives and lifestyles are strongly imbued by longstanding social, kinship and religious traditions as well as climatic and environmental conditions that influence the success or otherwise of harvests.

While coverage of medical care had been achieved through the establishment of health posts, and health centres throughout its districts, including rural areas, Malawi's mental health service was centralised and not at all integrated within primary health care (Udedi et al., 2013). Three mental health in-patient units housed around 600 beds in total, spread across the three regions—northern, central, and southern Malawi. There was minimal community mental health outreach work, and where they did exist, they were extensions from these centres (Kauye & Mafuta, 2006). Due to the huge demands of communicable diseases, and child and maternal health, the general health care work force at health posts and centres had limited capacity—and had very limited biomedical training—for identifying and managing mental health problems (Udedi, 2016). This scarcity of resource, coupled with the limited recognition of common mental health problems (depression and anxiety) as health concerns and high levels of stigma noted towards people suffering from mental health issues (Crabb et al., 2012) meant that such institutions cared for only a small fraction of people experiencing the most severe mental illness, often following criminal actions.

The expansion of such mental health awareness and capacity building of community mental health services was the main driver for the task-shifting project. However, viewed from the local community, this was a very different perspective of 'mental health care'. Issues described as mental health problems were not seen as any new form of 'illness' or challenge for society. Behaviour of individuals that appeared odd, out of kilter with society's norms, or deviant were not new phenomena. From the community's sense, understandings of causation, classification, and treatment of such 'distress without physical cause' was embedded in people's religious, social, and cultural context (Kleinman, 1980). The response offered would be mobilised through both kinship and social structures and in certain instances more formally through organisations such as African traditional religious practice, Christian churches, and mosques (Steinforth, 2009).

Such networks that sought to care for and manage the disruptions caused by such behaviour and distress were pluralistic and often blended and ranged from healing practices based on religious text and traditions to distinctive forms of personhood and agency that manifest from connections between a person's spiritual, social, and individual worlds (Kpanake, 2018). To be precise, it's not that there was a treatment 'gap'—only a 'biomedical treatment gap'. Indeed, frequent broadcast and print media reports on the activities of traditional healers and Christian healing ministries indicate an omnipresent discourse about 'mental illness' in everyday life in Malawi (Englund, 2011; Simwaka et al., 2007) and an almost universal provision, with reports of up to 80% of the population accessing traditional healers (Malawi Ministry of Health, 2005). Nevertheless, it was with this backdrop that the Malawi Ministry of Health initiated the task-shifting project to train village health workers as part of a strategic plan to develop community mental health care provision. Over the project, all 850 HSAs from across the 32 health centres in the district undertook a three-day introduction to 'mental health' course, or, as it was termed, 'working with people in distress'. In contrast to many subsequent task-shifting initiatives, in this project, village workers were not taught to diagnose mental illness, only to respond therapeutically to people's 'distress', including when someone is fearful, low in mood, suicidal or violent to others. A deliberately psychosocial rather than biomedical approach was offered, and the workers were encouraged to respond from the perspective that a person's 'health' is impaired and to use problem-solving approaches to respond and to signpost to health centres if additional support was required.

An analysis of the health workers' interventions revealed they delivered four types of intervention:

1. interventions to promote safety and reduce the risk of harm to self or others,
2. advising a health model to understand a person's distress,
3. providing psychological and emotional support through talking and practical help, and
4. promoting psychosocial support for people through families and the wider community.

In addition, the health workers utilised the same 'health' perspective of distress to engage with wider community at formal village meetings, health talks and public meetings and they established support groups for distressed people and their family and carers. In two years of the project over 43,000 people attended these events.

By the end of the project, it was clear that the health workers had created a new service offering a 'health' model to people in distress, optimising help-seeking, and operating practical, and person-centred support. The health worker-facilitated mental health promotion activities attracted many attendees and revealed the extensive reach that such workers have within their communities. However, while from a GMH and 'implementation science' perspective, the project demonstrated the ability to implement to scale an intervention that harnesses the health workers' motivation and knowledge of context to provide a mental health service at community level—with further work needed to increase workers' fidelity to a therapeutic model and to develop appropriate measurement of outcomes (Patel et al., 2012)—from the perspective of the researchers and health professionals on the ground, fundamental questions remained and further answers were required. The non-diagnostic and non-prescriptive approach adopted by the project did reflect an appreciation of the complexity of the task being 'shifted' onto the health workers within this pluralistic health environment and, as such, anticipated the appropriateness or otherwise of imposing essentially one (biomedical) lens through which distress is viewed. For there remained little known of exactly how acceptable these health worker interventions were within the community, including how the people in distress responded to them. Understanding the interactions between the health worker and patients from within the context of the complete 'healing system' (Kleinman, 1980) that included wider pluralistic provision, needed further exploration.

One particular finding, the way that health workers described a person's 'problem' in their health records, repeatedly seemed to focus on certain behaviours and situations and appeared to indicate how such problems were being discussed in their interactions. On the surface, the interventions reported, match that learned in the three-day training and those from psychosocial packages of care designed for other low-resource settings, such as offering individual psychological and emotional support and mobilising community psychosocial resources (Lund et al., 2015). However, descriptions of distressing emotions were found to be present in just 6% of records. At the same time while the health workers reported acknowledging people's differing causal attributions for their distress, and including bewitchment attributions within their formulations, exactly how these discussions steer towards the 'practical' and even 'credible' interventions that were claimed was not fully apparent. While some of these findings may have resulted from artefacts of the way the health workers recorded their entries (the limitation of relatively perfunctory survey-type data), it nevertheless indicated the need to explore these types of interactions further. How were the health workers helping? For the way in which the health workers and people in distress interact, and the relationship that is co-created between them, provides a frame from which to understand both the complexity of the pluralistic health landscape and the mental health role of the health workers. To pursue this, a further qualitative study explored how both the health workers and their patients viewed the nature and causes of 'distress' and revealed a much more nuanced picture of how distress was perceived, attributed, and responded to (Wright & Maliwichi-Senganimalunje, 2020).

Firstly, shifts in the language used to describe the difficulties were detected. While not entirely unacceptable to patients and carers, the psychosocial causation of mental illness was nevertheless introducing a 'health/illness' model into situations previously considered a part of life. As described in Chap. 2, the shift in the conception from *kukumudwa* (a severe yet sane reaction to life's hardships) to *nkhawa* (low mood/despair and potentially a precursor to 'madness' or *misala*) indicated a subtle modification towards a medicalisation of life (Summerfield, 2008). Similarly, the view of drug or alcohol dependency as an illness was being introduced where previously the community tended to assert moral judgement over how a person was expected to deal with life problems (Fig. 4.1).

Secondly, the study revealed that traditional medicine was regarded as an 'open secret' since the majority of patients (and many health workers) used the services of traditional healers. The privileging of biomedicine at health centres meant that patients were reluctant to disclose their use of traditional medicine to health centre staff and where this had been disclosed to health workers, they responded by discrediting traditional medicine and promoting biomedical understandings. This created tensions for health workers and patients in their discussions of their distress and treatment responses. Indeed, the study exposed the dilemma that such medical pluralism raised for those working in the health care system. The task-shifting approach and work of the village health workers had impacted on the way mental health is perceived by privileging a 'biopsychosocial' understanding of distress that incorporated the indigenous understanding that people react to stressful environments (*kukumudwa*). While

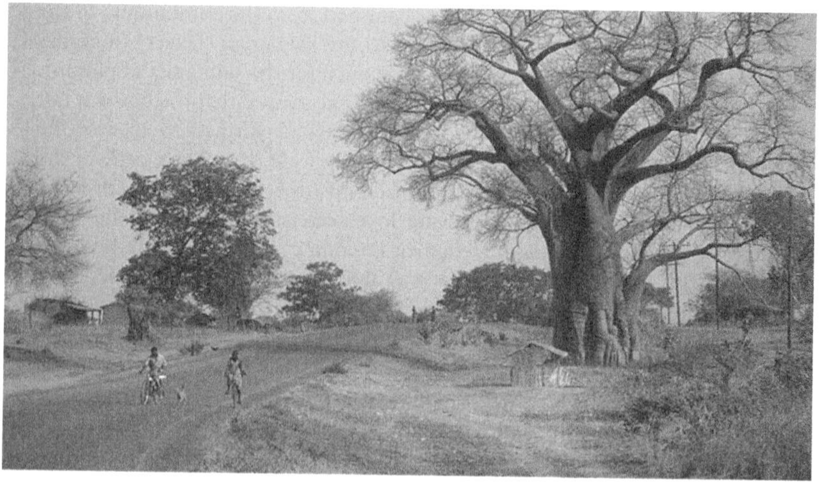

Fig. 4.1 Rural Southern Malawi. (Photo: Steph Common, 2013)

compelling for many, it did not inform any drive for integration with other healing systems (Musyimi et al., 2016). Instead, it appears to have reinforced the demarcation of the biomedical from traditional health systems (Kottai & Ranganathan, 2020) whereby the health workers and patients navigate around the two parallel systems, rather than to explore or negotiate different meanings. So, while the project can be said to have integrated mental health into primary care, it certainly did not integrate within the wider helping system. A case example from fieldwork illustrates the kind of complex interactions that occur in a pluralistic health environment.

> A 14-year-old boy recently became disturbed and violent – damaging a market stall and threatening people. People in the village were becoming alarmed by his unpredictable behaviour and, suspecting he may have been 'bewitched', suggested his uncle takes him to consult a traditional herbalist. The uncle considered the boy had a mental illness and was very uncertain that the consultation would help. However, not taking the boy to the herbalist risked him being seen as neglecting the boy's (and the community's) best interests which would lead to social disapproval. Also, because certain members of the community had started to accuse the boy of being a maleficent 'wizard' (rather than the victim of witchcraft), ascertaining the specific nature of the spiritual explanation through the opinion of the traditional herbalist was vital since the latter accusation might lead to the boy being

subjected to serious physical harm or banished from the community. In the event, the uncle accompanied the boy to the sing'anga (healer), together with several elders of the community (to vouch for the sing'anga's opinion), and following a short consultation, received the avowal that the boy was not a wizard but had been bewitched. A ritual was performed to appease the family spirits, who had been agitated by an episode of violence early in the boy's life, and the boy was accepted back into the community, with community members vowing to provide love, care and security to the boy. Whilst expressing scepticism whether attending the traditional herbalist would help, the uncle nevertheless was able to secure the boy's safety and care and his own status within the community.

Wright and Maliwichi-Senganimalunje (2020, pp. 41–42).

Outside of the biomedical health service, the uncle sourced what became a life-saving intervention from the *sing'anga*, whose formulation informed an understanding of the boy's experience of distress, alongside past traumatic events in the family, and procured a resolution that allayed the fears of the community. The belief that ancestors exert an influence over living relatives is embedded in the community and provides meaning to otherwise inexplicable events (van Breugel, 2001; Tobert, 2017). Whatever accompanying social welfare or biomedical interventions, the boy's health could not have been safeguarded without reference to such conceptions.

Despite the expediential growth of task-shifting initiatives with non-specialist workers in the last decade and even the claim that within the task-shifting projects, traditional modalities of healing involving the family, social normalisation and spiritual approaches are being acknowledged (Whitley, 2015), this appears far from the reality. Several fated attempts at collaboration between biomedical and traditional healing approaches have been documented (Davar, 2014; Musyimi et al., 2016; Sood, 2016; Akol et al., 2018; Herman et al., 2018; Solera-Deuchar et al., 2020) and found that this contested space between formal (usually biomedical) and informal (lay) care systems leads invariably to the side-lining of traditional understandings and approaches and the attempted co-option of traditional workers to the biomedical 'cause' of identifying people with 'mental illness'. Kottai and Ranganathan (2020) have pointed to the way that such task-shifting approaches reshape 'suffering' as a brain disorder. Alternative culturally attuned understandings are side-lined by essentialist thinking dominated by biomedicine, with an accompanying disrespect and discrediting of traditional healing approaches. The socio-cultural approach to psychology proposed by Markus and Hamedani at the start of this chapter sees cultural meanings and practices not as phenomena that operate outside us as individuals and to which we relate, but as aspects of our internal world that inform the way we think and the lens through which we understand and experience life (Markus & Hamedani, 2007). Such a proposition renders problematic attempts to assert one particular way of understanding and responding to something as nuanced and socially constructed as 'distress' (Horwitz, 2003). On the contrary when considering therapeutic responses, aligning perspectives of patients and providers creates a framework of trust and positive expectancy that potentiates positive outcomes (Asay & Lambert, 1999). All factors are culturally interwoven.

Lastly, and most interestingly when it comes to appreciating the dynamic nature of knowledge and how people navigate different types of knowledge, the health workers appeared to show a particular response to the biomedical dominance. When examining the way that the three most prominent interventions were deployed, it became clear that workers attuned their interventions to the cultural framework of their patients so that 'practical help' called on traditional village structures of patronage and obligation, 'counselling' was delivered, not as a structured, unconditional, and person-centred approach (as taught in trainings), but as an opportunity for regaining 'personhood' and their role in the community, and 'support groups' enacted the value of both providing and receiving support within a collectivist culture. It appeared that the psychosocial interventions taught and delivered through the project were being re-contextualised within *umunthu* philosophy rather than the psychosocial frame described by biomedicine. The rich indigenous cultural philosophy of *umunthu* that underpins everyday life in rural Malawi presented a dilemma for the health workers in their delivery of interventions. In response, and under both the gaze and the guise of biomedicine, the health workers navigated between biomedical understandings of mental illness and traditional African understandings to fashion supportive interventions that were attuned to their cultural norms. Such a standpoint positions the health workers' adapted interventions as a form of resistance to a dominant epistemology and from which alternative understandings and responses to distress are being generated.

These findings from Malawi provide contemporary empirical evidence of not only the privileging of certain knowledge and the subsuming of others, but also how different actors adapt and respond in this environment—patients, health workers and mental health professionals. A similar thread is found in the work of Mills and Lacroix (2019) who, in different 'mental health gap' training initiatives, including in India and West Africa, reported how local epistemologies of distress interrupted or resisted the universalised knowledge and 'tools' advocated in training. The continued dominance of biomedicine within the formal health care sector, in the face of manifest pluralistic understandings within communities' informal care and traditional health care systems, is indicative of the colonial endeavour by representing the explicit hierarchy of Western over non-Western knowledge systems (Ibrahim, 2014: Fernando, 2014) and rendering powerless indigenous understandings such as the role of ***umunthu*** in fostering mental health in Malawi. The impact on people experiencing psychological distress is a continued dislocation of formal from informal mental health care and help-seeking.

Whilst what drives the GMH's universalistic assumptions about effective responses to distress can clearly be described as a type of colonial enterprise, the explanation for why local health workers act in this way is equally revealing. Mills (2014) speaks of the 'pretending' of patients confronted with the power of the psychiatric gaze—and links this to the mimicry and subversion of the colonised. Perhaps the same is happening here for the health workers in Malawi? They are operating a 'sly normalisation' and 'invisibility', whereby what are heralded as biomedical interventions are in fact the delivery of culturally embedded therapeutic approaches. For the health workers, practical help was marshalled through traditional structures, counselling became advice to provide the person with hope and a steer, and support groups became more than providing a safe place for emotional exchange, to a forum for the enactment of values, reflection, and reinforcement of ***umunthu***, of positive social capital and obligation. These studies therefore add important empirical evidence to the emerging critique of the pedagogy of mental health task-shifting and related approaches in international contexts (Mills & Lacroix, 2019; Mills & Hilberg, 2019; Read, 2019) by bringing to light the experiences of different actors.

A further technique, realised from colonial governance practice, is the insidious system of identifying and 'training' local 'interpreters'—in this case mental health professionals and education systems –trained to maintain the authority of Western dominance (Mills, 2014; Wright & Jayawickrama, 2021). Within otherwise depleted health sectors, the status afforded such 'interpreters'—alongside the continued financial support through GMH projects—protects and sustains this one biomedical approach to 'managing' distress, regardless of context and indigenous knowledges. Indeed, much of this is an echo of voices from the field of global health outside of mental health where 'travelling models' bear no semblance to the socio-cultural context of the health workers and system (Olivier de Sardan et al., 2017). Not just ethically dubious, but also ineffective, Olivier De Sardan's critique extends to the whole development project where criticism is withheld in the unequal relationship between donor and recipient (Ridde & Olivier De Sardan, 2022)—surely the embodiment of colonialism?

4.3 The 2004 Tsunami in Sri Lanka and Mental Health Interventions

> In the Southern district of Galle, a foreign volunteer team dressed in bright yellow t-shirts and matching caps entered a temporary accommodation campsite, which housed over 100 Tsunami-affected families. The team, travelling in a hired bus decorated with bright yellow banners and streamers, looked like a troop from a Brazilian Mardi Gras parade. They then proceeded to hastily mobilize the transit camp authorities to round up the children for what they termed 'psychosocial therapy'. Bright-coloured tents were quickly assembled in the camps. The resident children, with a mixture of both amusement and confusion, complied with the instructions from their bemused elders, and were soon shuffled into groups, according to age. The foreign teams then began massaging (using an ointment) the limbs and foreheads of these 'traumatized children', all in the name of 'psychosocial healing and therapy'. In one instance a masseur, who spoke English as a second language, was applying Betadine (an antiseptic) on the face of a young boy who had no apparent cuts or abrasions on his face … A World Health Organization (WHO) team visiting the camp to conduct an initial assessment witnessed this 'psychosocial' phenomenon and reported it to the relevant district level health authorities.
>
> Observed at a post-tsunami displacement camp in Sri Lanka
> (Quoted in Wickramage, 2006, p. 164).

An extremely powerful earthquake rocked northern Indonesia on Sunday 26 December 2004, which sent massive tsunamis crashing into several countries, including Sri Lanka. The U.S. Geological Survey reported a quake of magnitude 9, which struck at 8 a.m. about 100 miles off the west coast of the island of Sumatra. Massive tsunamis stemming from the Sumatra epicentre hit Sri Lanka—some 1000 miles west in the Indian Ocean—creating the worst natural hazard in the recent history of

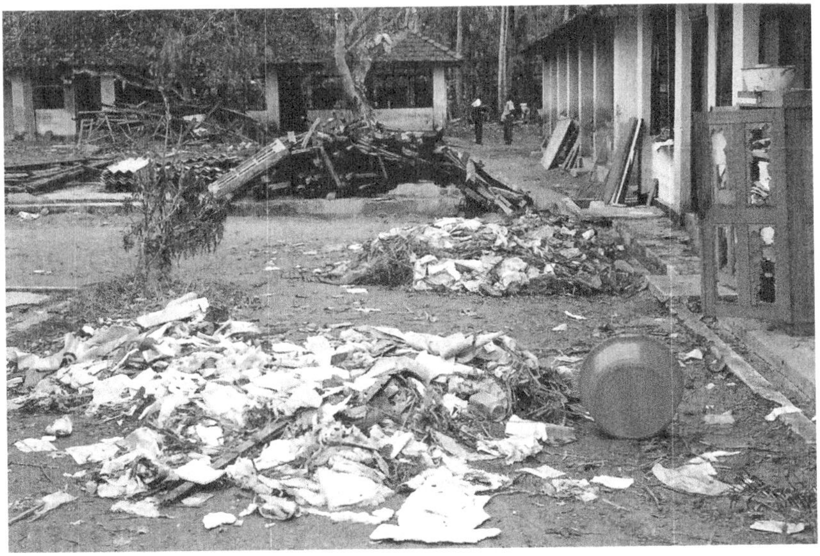

Fig. 4.2 Tsunami Impact in a Southern Sri Lankan School. (Photo: Janaka Jayawickrama (2004))

Sri Lanka. This is the largest earthquake on Earth since the 9.2-magnitude Good Friday Earthquake, which struck Alaska, USA, on 27 March 1964, and the fourth largest since 1900 (USGS, 2018) (Fig. 4.2).

The multiple tsunamis which struck and ravaged coastal regions all over the Indian Ocean devastated regions including the Indonesian province of Aceh, the coast of Sri Lanka, coastal areas of the Indian state of Tamil Nadu, the resort island of Phuket, Thailand, and even as far away as Somalia and several other countries in Africa, 4500 km (2800 mi) or more west of the epicentre (USGS, 2018). In the first four weeks after the tsunami, the Sri Lankan population that were not affected by the disaster helped the affected community (Jayawickrama, 2004). Then, the international humanitarian agencies started to flood the country, bringing what might be described as another tsunami upon the affected communities. This also prompted humanitarian agencies to divert major resources and personnel to promote programmes in keeping with dominant Western concepts of "mental health programmes".

This emphasis of mental health—by both international and local non-governmental organisations (NGOs)—based on Western-style counselling, psychotherapy, and befriending was at the expense of programmes addressing the physical destruction wrought by the tsunami. Many individuals from Europe and North America proclaiming themselves as "clinicians", "certified psychologists," and "mental health professionals" started to conduct their own interventions without any international or local supervision.

> He came into our village after the tsunami with an assistant. We were told [by the local NGO] that he is a mental health expert from the UK. They said that they are going to treat us with our mental health problems. Then this man sat down in front of my wife and started pointing a finger at her eyes. Yes, we are sad and upset about all what happen. I thought that they are going to help us to re-build our lives, but I got really mad when I saw this strange man pointing a finger at my wife. When I questioned this in an angry tone, the translator said that my anger is the mental health problem, and I need special support. What nonsense? I asked them to leave my place immediately.
>
> A fisherman from tsunami-affected Eastern Sri Lanka
> Direct discussion with the Author, October 2005
> (Quoted in Jayawickrama (2009, pp. 8–9)).

Not only were these 'experts' conducting interventions without supervision and labelling the affected population with "trauma", "depression", and "anxiety" diagnoses, but they also disregarded community concerns.

> One morning a team of 'psychosocial specialists' came to our camp. We were told that they are from the US and here to help us to provide psychosocial activities. All of us gathered in the community hall and through translation they told us the importance of sharing our sadness and grief about our losses from the tsunami. Then the man and the woman who came from the US started hugging us. I felt very uncomfortable and irritated. During the tea break I went home and told my mother, and she told me to keep away from them.
>
> A teenage girl from tsunami-affected Eastern Sri Lanka
> Direct discussion with the author, October 2005
> (Quoted in Jayawickrama (2009, p. 9)).

What became apparent was not only the "clinicians'" or "mental health professionals'" lack of appropriate qualifications or capacity to work with tsunami-affected communities, but that they were working with communities without any appreciation of local cultural norms, values, and practices. In one instance, the first author of this book, who was coordinating the national response, met with a "clinical psychologist" from the USA, who wanted to devise a national trauma programme. After much discussion and requests, she revealed that she was an educational psychologist without a license to even practise in the US. Many of these external mental health experts were also conducting trainings and workshops for staff members of local organisations that had for decades been assisting the conflict-affected communities, and yet were still not humble enough to receive feedback.

> The workshop was filled with presentations and should have [been] done in a more participatory manner. I don't think that one could become really qualified to implement even parts of these guidelines after a two days' workshop. Also, they expect us to give feedback about the effectiveness about these guidelines within two or three months. Well, this is too much pressure and rushing. There were no discussions per say about how Sri Lanka could adopt these guidelines into local realities. Then the workshops they conducted in local languages had so many errors with bad translations. I think that this will not produce anything effective as there is no support mechanism in Sri Lanka to assist field level problems and I am not aware about any monitoring process.
>
> A Sri Lankan UN staff member that works on mental health
> Direct discussion with the Author, March 2007
> (Quoted in Jayawickrama (2009, p. 12)).

Further, many of these mental health interventions did not have any idea what the affected populations were requesting. There was clearly a mismatch of expectations, and yet, the international "mental health experts" were determined to achieve their targets.

> The foreigner who came to our camp asked all of us to list down our problems after the tsunami. We listed things like schools, education, housing, and difficulties in this camp. After listening to us he said that we have mental problems as we do not want to discuss our feelings. He wanted to us to talk about our mental problems. We could not understand any of that and we left the foreigner and his workshop.
>
> Teenage girl from Tsunami-affected Western Province in Sri Lanka
> Direct discussion with the Author, March 2005
> (Quoted in Jayawickrama (2009, p. 13))

One Canadian artist, who had been collaborating with Sri Lankan practitioners in the previous months, observed this chaotic drama.

> Teams of zealous professional traumatologists are descending on a regular basis from Manhattan to Mattakalappu [Batticaloa in Eastern Sri Lanka]. They have acquired their peerless, state-of-the-art trauma counseling experience during 9/11 so they're the world's best and they've come in their mercy to bring treatment and consolation to people in the refugee camps. ... If the traumatologist can tap dance, juggle watermelons, balance a jug of lemonade on her nose and do some serious hugging or look-into-my-eyes-darling therapy while perched on the table performing, she will win the day!
> Hogan (2005), Batticaloa Butterfly Peace Garden
> Tsunami Report – Z Doc 1, 5 May 2005

Summerfield (1999) has explained a common occurrence where the international agencies and experts expect disaster-affected people to have emotional problems and not practical problems. So, without understanding the social, political, cultural, economic, and environmental realities of the community, these international agencies and mental health experts were assuming that there was a "mental health" problem. This exposes a huge gap in understanding the requirement for mental health interventions during the tsunami response in Sri Lanka. According to Euro-North American tradition of biomedical experts such as Brier (2004) and Kessler et al. (1995), disasters and conflicts represent a set of traumatic events that increase the prevalence of mental disorders. In this argument, the overall epidemiology of trauma, depression, and anxiety is considered significant and requiring of treatments. Alternatively, local attributions formulate people's worldview regarding disasters and catastrophes in relation to an understanding of their religions, cultures, and traditions. This medicalised labelling of mental health can be seen to ignore people's own capacities; their relationships, kinships (affinities and blood ties), and to undercut wider socio-cultural, political, and economic, capabilities (Summerfield & Hume, 1992). In this way, Jayawickrama (2010), Summerfield and Hume (1992) and Summerfield and Toser (1991) have argued that medical models do not represent a socialised view of mental health. Experiences of massive catastrophes such as a tsunami or other forms of danger and their aftermath in societies such as Sri Lanka are not individualised experiences, but instead, happen within social settings. Those who need assistance reveal themselves and the process that determines how victims become survivors (as the majority do) are played out over time. Jones (2004) a child psychiatrist from the UK, reflected upon her experiences with Serbian and Muslim young people during the Bosnian War in the 1990s,

> [A]fter meeting children in Gorazde [a municipality in Bosnia and Herzegovina] I came to believe that humanitarian programmes and mental health professionals were approaching the subject of war trauma from the wrong direction.
>
> Jones (2004, p. 4).

Scholars such as Kleinman (2006), Korn (1997), and Summerfield (1999) argue that most crisis-affected populations are optimistically dealing with dangers of life without outside expert help. As we saw after the tsunami in Sri Lanka, it was local people that provided the initial response. So, while certainly there are mental health and wellbeing related issues that face the affected populations, and outsiders to the community may look to a medical response, the insider experience is of ancient wisdoms, traditional knowledge, religions, and cultures that are addressing the challenges related to crises in a pragmatic manner (Jayawickrama, 2010). The Tsunami Evaluation Coalition's joint evaluation of the international response to the Indian Ocean tsunami in all affected countries (Cosgrave, 2007, p. 4), presents a set of findings that points to the importance of local or insider tenue:

1. It was local people themselves who provided almost all immediate life-saving action and the early emergency support, as is commonly the case in disasters. The TEC studies found that international agencies experienced major problems in scaling up their own responses. Pre-existing links, and mutual respect, between international agencies and local partners also led to better use of both international and local capacities.
2. International action was most effective when enabling, facilitating, and supporting local actors. International agencies often brushed local capacities aside, even though they subscribe to norms and standards that call for engagement with and accountability to local actors such as governments, communities, and local NGOs. International agencies often ignored local structures and did not

communicate well with local communities nor hold themselves accountable to them.
3. There were many examples of poor-quality work in the response to the tsunami, not only in the relief phase (largely from inexperienced agencies) but also in the recovery phase.
4. The tsunami highlighted the arbitrary nature of the current funding system for humanitarian emergencies. This system produces an uneven and unfair flow of funds for emergencies that encourages neither investment in capacity nor responses that are proportionate to need.

The tsunami experience of Sri Lanka suggests that uncertainty and dangers are not extraordinary and short-lived events but sit within the ongoing context of peoples' lives. Jayawickrama (2010, p. 116) documented the insider or community learning and responses to the tsunami in Batticaloa of Eastern Sri Lanka:

1. Uncertainty and dangers are part of life. Suffering is part of being human.
2. Importance of family and community.
3. Value of religion.
4. Ownership and responsibility of interventions.
5. Helplessness and powerlessness.
6. Sadness and desperation.
7. Worries about the future.
8. Lack of freedom (due to the impact of the civil war in the area, which ended in 2009).
   Jayawickrama (2010, p. 116).

This research strongly suggests that the community draws on traditional and cultural mechanisms in dealing with suffering and uncertainty and to address danger, as well as to improve wellbeing. Their worries, hopes, dreams, and aspirations are positively and negatively affecting their mental health and wellbeing in terms of past, present, and future. A separate process has been established by the community to re-convey ownership of their lives and their more in-depth issues, and towards finding solutions. What emerges from the Sri Lankan experience of the tsunami was that communities consider suffering through crises to be part of being human. They deal with these suffering by using religion, culture, traditional knowledge, and ancient wisdoms, and receive practical support from their families, friends, and communities to do so (Jayawickrama, 2010). However, the problem was and is that the international mental health interventions reroute the focus away from the way the affected populations view their major problems and challenges. When someone is hungry, or needing shelter, and have lost their loved ones and all their properties, they need practical help, not someone to talk about it.

Arnold (1988) and Headrick (1981) have argued that medical approaches and systems introduced by imperial forces in non-Western societies were a tool of political, economic, social, and cultural domination. In the same way, the mental health experts that arrived in Sri Lanka during 1990s can be seen as responding to political and economic needs of global capitalism. In fulfilling the needs of the capital marketplace, there was no interest or effort to understand the wants and needs of the affected populations. As one farmer from conflict-affected Sri Lanka in 2005 put it (quoted in Jayawickrama, 2013, p. 31), the researchers and experts were only interested in gathering information, perhaps for their valued research publications.

> No one within our community requested these international organisations to come and help us. We have been surviving the conflict since 1980s and disasters since 1950s. Before 1990, we were helping each other and the few organisations in our area were listening to us. Now, it is different – all these foreigners and their assistant Sri Lankans who comes in Land Cruisers with questionnaires only want our information. Then they disappear and a new group comes. I think that if they can't do any good, they shouldn't come.

However, despite this backdrop, a different approach was taken by a collaborative effort in Sri Lanka. In 1994 a combined team from McMaster University's Centre for International Health and the Spiral Garden[1] visited Batticaloa in Eastern Sri Lanka and began working with a Jesuit priest born and bred in Batticaloa, and a noted environmentalist who had already been working in Batticaloa for many years. The result was the Butterfly Peace Garden, which opened its doors in 1996. Between its inception and 2002, over 600 schoolchildren, from 20 communities around Batticaloa, representing local ethnic groups attended its programmes (Chase & Bush, 2002). At the time the Garden was established as the main focus of

[1]The Spiral Garden at the Hugh MacMillan Rehabilitation Centre (now Holland Bloorview Kids Rehabilitation Hospital) for physically challenged children was co-founded by the Canadian artist Paul Hogan in 1983.

government and non-governmental intervention in Batticaloa to meet basic food, shelter, and physical needs, as the understanding at that time was when the physical needs of people are met, they themselves are capable of dealing with their mental and spiritual needs. In that, the local churches, Hindu temples, and Muslim mosques played a significant role. However, the Garden allowed children's expressiveness to take the lead in ways that the narrowly mandated, prescribed, and short-term focused approaches of government and non-governmental organizations did not (Lawrence, 2003, p. 4). The approach of the Garden acknowledged that despite the fact that the children may be young, and may have suffered the devastating effects of conflict, they can still be agents for change—both within themselves and within the wider community:

> Both those aspects of the child which are wounded and those which remain resilient are addressed. By tending to the garden within the human heart as well as the outer garden of earthly experience with equal imagination and compassion, children can heal and become healers within their communities.
>
> Chase and Bush (2002, p. 6).

The methodology of the Garden which continues to today, is "presence (mindfulness) in poiesis (the creative flow of imagination) as the practice of peace (balance between inner and outer)" (Lawrence, 2003, p. 2). The Garden believes that the 'river of poiesis' is reached through ritual, play, and silence. The Garden Path practice evolved through a process of adoption from other cultures (such as native North America, Aboriginal culture in Australia, and various parts of Asia), adaptation, and inculturation, that is, "made relevant to the Batticaloa Garden in ways specifically appropriate to the variables and conditions found there" (Lawrence, 2003, p. 32). Over the years, the Garden Path has been created and supported by many different organisations and individuals from different cultures, countries, races, ethnic groups, ages, genders, and religions (Lawrence, 2003; Chase & Bush, 2002).

> This oasis of imagination and creativity brings together animation artists, peace-workers, ritual healers and children from various ethnic and religious groups, joining hands, hearts and minds to nourish the spirit of healing and peace for generations to come in Sri Lanka.
>
> Children and animators of the Butterfly Garden, as collected and retold in English by Paul Hogan (1997, p. 6).

In response to an endless stream of journalists, traumatologists, wannabe researchers, videographers, apocalyptic tourists, and diplomatic do-gooders visiting the Garden, a Foreign Policy Green Paper (The Butterfly Peace Garden, 2000), was drafted to protect the community and its members from the impacts of such exposures. The Green Paper provides clear guidance on establishing relations with outsiders in terms of assessing potential collaborators as well as the types of relationships that the Butterfly Peace Garden may expect to enter into. Potential outside collaborators (whether Sri Lankan or international) must satisfy the Garden by answering a number of questions in order to demonstrate their integrity (amongst other things). As an absolute minimum, potential collaborators must be able to answer 'yes' to the following crucial question:

> Is this in the best interests of the children?
> Butterfly Peace Garden (2000, p. 1).

By the time of the 2004 tsunami, the Butterfly Peace Garden and related activities had been in Batticaloa for over ten years. However, the 'external' agencies that arrived after the tsunami paid little or no attention to what was available locally. Instead, of collaborating with local populations and groups in building support, services, and responses, they assumed the affected Sri Lankan populations were 'traumatised' and as such they prescribed and implemented culturally inappropriate and often harmful interventions to deal with psychological distress without understanding any local realities.

4.4 Global Mental Health Within the Capitalist Marketplace

All mainstream disciplines and human activities, including mental health, have emerged, developed, and operate within globalised social, economic, and political contexts. The neglect of these contexts by mental health professionals and organisations, especially considering what might be seen as their role in oppression within the capitalist marketplace, has been one of the ignored and hidden threats to people's health. For this capitalist marketplace is itself an extension of coloniality.

The colonial project is often narrowly defined as operating in certain geographic areas and at certain historical periods and that the project is no longer functioning in the world. Indeed, many in former colonies believed that once the colonisers had left the people would be able to move forward unhindered to enjoy the freedoms of development. This was not so.

In many former colonies, the colonial project left behind not only social, political, cultural, and economic structures, but also 'scientific' and intellectual legacies. Both in Sri Lanka and in Malawi, where there had always been medical pluralism, living and working in a system dominated by biomedicine upholds a neoliberalism and capital market ethos and reflects a colonialism of thinking whereby alternative perspectives are silenced (epistemic injustice) and alternative practices denigrated (oppression). As a result, there are many 'interpreters' and few 'resisters'!

Since assumptions of the superiority of Western biomedical thinking are mainstream across education and health services in postcolonial countries, there are few examples where such hegemony is resisted, and alternative indigenous models openly pushback. One such novel example of curriculum development in Malawian medical education (Bandawe, 2005) offers an insight into the penetration of Western-based thinking into the mind and attitudes of intelligent young Malawians. Bandawe states:

> The next step in the evolution of the course was to introduce a topic explicitly grounded in an African philosophy to which Malawians could relate. Thus, in 2003, I introduced a topic for the first years entitled 'uMunthology'. When I first pronounced this name in class, one of the students remarked out loud in the vernacular: 'I hope, sir, you are not taking us for a ride'. The remark is telling. There would be no questioning of such a topic if it were imported from the West, but a Malawian topic caused students to immediately doubt its authenticity. So instilled is the Western-based model of education that liberating the minds of students is an ongoing process.
>
> Bandawe (2005, p. 296)

After the tsunami in Sri Lanka, the international mental health interventions created two main challenges. Firstly, the mental health projects took away much needed financial assistance within the humanitarian response and rebuilding process. Secondly, these international mental health interventions attempted to create a political economy, which was not common to the affected populations. Both these challenges were attempting to facilitate a new market, a new market of "mental health" where there are "professionals" that are selling a service, and "consumers" that are buying that service. This is disaster capitalism (Klein, 2007). In response, local communities including many faith communities in tsunami- and conflict-affected Sri Lanka decided to conduct their own interventions to improve wellbeing. Such religious and social knowledge systems acted as vehicles for such resistance and many rural communities that had been affected by the tsunami in 2004 chose to follow traditional practices to improve their mental health instead of attending psychological clinics or psychosocial programmes.

In Malawi, the GMH movement has been "educating" the local professionals to raise awareness and conduct therapeutic interventions. Although the challenges in Malawi can be labelled more as developmental than crisis induced, the humanitarian impact is equally profound. When people have no access to food, clean water, housing, education, and health services, the role of mental health becomes a diversion from the real developmental challenges. Even while this diversion creates "good business" for the GMH project, local people resist this through their engagement with traditional systems of healing, and the local health workers adapt their interventions from the original training intention to an understanding that is more plausible to the recipients of such care. So, within such a landscape, in reality, from a biomedical perspective, what is planned is often not what is delivered. In the face of the inadequacies of response to people's suffering, local health workers resist the confines of the biomedical approach by creating opportunities to extend the scope of their interventions to user-centred advocacy and more socially orientated interventions. Thus, where the individualism of mental illness diverts attention from structural deficits and the violence of colonialism seen in the reaction of health workers from Malawi and Sri Lanka reveal a sometimes hidden, but nonetheless vibrant resistance to psychiatrisation (Logan & Karter, 2022). Before we develop our discussion in Chap. 6 of the ways in which people's experiences of distress can be responded to beyond these colonial approaches, we will first progress our epistemic disobedience by exploring the extent to which such biomedical hegemony concerning mental health and its resistance may be operating in the UK. Chapter 5 will help us to explore whether the same notions of coloniality and expressions of power through the medicalisation and individualisation of distress are not present in the seat of colonial power itself.

References

Akol, A., Moland, K. M., Babirye, J. N., & Engebretsen, I. M. S. (2018). "We are like co-wives": Traditional healers' views on collaborating with the formal child and adolescent mental health system in Uganda. *BMC Health Services Research, 18*, 1–9.

Arnold, D. (1988). Introduction: Disease, medicine and empire. In D. Arnold (Ed.), *Imperial medicine and indigenous societies* (pp. 1–26). Manchester University Press.

Asay, T. P., & Lambert, M. J. (1999). The empirical case for the common factors in therapy: Quantitative findings. In M. A. Hubble, B. L. Duncan, & S. D. Miller (Eds.), *The heart and soul of change: What works in therapy* (pp. 23–55). American Psychological Association.

Bandawe, C. (2005). Psychology brewed in an African pot: Indigenous philosophies and the quest for relevance. *Higher Education Policy, 18*, 289–300.

Brier, J. (2004). *Psychological assessment of adult posttraumatic states: Phenomenology, diagnosis, and measurement* (2nd ed.). American Psychological Association.

Butterfly Peace Garden. (2000). *Green paper: Towards a foreign policy for the democratic anarchy of the butterfly peace garden of Batticaloa*. BPG.

Chase, R., & Bush, K. (2002). The mental health of war affected children: A community-based rehabilitation and reconciliation program. Sri Lanka's Eastern Province. *Asia Pacific Journal on Disability and Rehabilitation, 2*, 50–66.

Cosgrave, J. (2007). Tsunami evaluation coalition: Synthesis report: Expanded summary. Joint evaluation of the international response to the Indian Ocean tsunami. *TEC–Tsunami Evaluation Coalition.*

Crabb, J., Stewart, R. C., Kokota, D., Masson, N., Chabunya, S., & Krishnadas, R. (2012). Attitudes towards mental illness in Malawi: A cross-sectional survey. *BMC Public Health, 12*, 1–6.

Davar, B. C. (2014). Globalizing psychiatry and the case of 'vanishing' alternatives in a neocolonial state. *Disability and the Global South, 1*(2), 266–284.

Englund, H. (2011). *Human rights and African airwaves*. Indiana University Press.

Fernando, S. (2014). *Mental health worldwide: Culture, globalization and development*. Palgrave Macmillan.

Headrick, D. R. (1981). *The tools of empire: Technology and European imperialism in the nineteenth century*. Oxford University Press.

Herman, A. R., Pullen, S. J., Lange, B. C. L., Christian-Brathwaite, N., Ulloa, M., Kempeh, M., Karnga, M., Johnson, D., Harris, B., Henderson, D. C., & Borba, C. P. C. (2018). Closing the mental health treatment gap through the collaboration of traditional and Western medicine in Liberia. *International Journal of Culture and Mental Health, 11*(4), 693–704.

Hogan, P. (1997). *The butterfly peace garden: Children and animators of the butterfly garden*. As collected and retold in English by Paul Hogan, (1997), Blood of the mango and other tales from the Butterfly Garden of Batticaloa.

Hogan, P. (2005). *Batticaloa butterfly peace garden: Tsunami report—Z doc 1*. The Butterfly Peace Garden.

Horwitz, A. V. (2003). *Creating mental illness*. University of Chicago Press.

Ibrahim, M. (2014). Mental health in Kenya: Not yet Uhuru. *Disability and the Global South, 1*(2), 393–400.

Jayawickrama, J. (2004). *Portrait of a disaster: Rapid assessment report of the effects of tsunami crushes in Sri Lanka*. Disaster Management and Information Programme (DMIP).

Jayawickrama, J. (2009). Ethical thinking: International mental health activities and communities, summer issue. *Fourth World Journal, 8*(1), 6–18.

Jayawickrama. J. (2010). *Rethinking mental health and wellbeing interventions in disaster and conflict affected communities: Case studies from Sri Lanka, Sudan and Malawi*. PhD thesis, Northumbria University.

Jayawickrama, J. (2013). 'If they can't do any good, they shouldn't come': Northern evaluators in southern realities. *Journal of Peacebuilding & Development, 8*(2), 26–41.

Jones, L. (2004). *Then they started shooting: Growing up in wartime Bosnia*. Harvard University Press.

Kauye, F., & Mafuta, C. (2006). Country profile: Malawi. *International Psychiatry, 4*, 9–11.

Kessler, R. C., Sonnega, A., Bromet, E., Hughes, M., & Nelson, C. B. (1995). Post-traumatic stress disorder in the National Comorbidity Survey. *Archives of General Psychiatry, 52*, 1048–1060.

Klein, N. (2007). *The shock doctrine: The rise of disaster capitalism*. Macmillan.

Kleinman, A. (1980). *Patients and healers in the context of culture: An exploration of the borderland between anthropology, medicine and psychiatry*. University of California Press.

Kleinman, A. (2006). *What really matters: Living a moral life amidst uncertainty and danger*. Oxford University Press.

Korn, L. (1997). *Community trauma and development: Imposed development undermines the individual spirit and traumatizes the community*. The World Conference on Violence and Human Coexistence, University College, Dublin and the Center for World Indigenous Studies. U.S.A, Dublin: Ireland.

Kottai, S. R., & Ranganathan, S. (2020). Task-shifting in community mental health in Kerala: Tensions and ruptures. *Medical Anthropology, 39*(6), 538–552.

Kpanake, L. (2018). Cultural concepts of the person and mental health in Africa. *Transcultural Psychiatry, 55*(2), 198–218.

Lawrence, P. (2003). *The ocean of stories: Children's imagination, creativity, and reconciliation in eastern Sri Lanka*. International Centre for Ethnic Studies.

Logan, J., & Karter, J. M. (2022). Psychiatrization of resistance: The co-option of consumer, survivor, and ex-patient movements in the global south. *Frontiers in Sociology, 7*, 784390.

Lund, C., Tomlinson, M., & Patel, V. (2015). Integration of mental health into primary care in low-income and middle-income countries: The PRIME mental healthcare plans. *British Journal of Psychiatry*, s1–s3.

Malawi Ministry of Health. (2005). *Emergency obstetrics care services in Malawi. Report of a nationwide assessment*. MoH.

Markus, H. R., & Hamedani, M. Y. G. (2007). Sociocultural psychology: The dynamic interdependence among self-systems and social systems. In H. Kitayama & D. Cohen (Eds.), *Handbook of cultural psychology*. Guilford Press.

Mills, C. (2014). *Decolonizing global mental health: The psychiatrization of the majority world*. Routledge.

Mills, C., & Hilberg, E. (2019). 'Built for expansion': The 'social life' of the WHO's mental health GAP intervention guide. *Sociology of Health and Illness, 41*(S1), 162–175.

Mills, C., & Lacroix, K. (2019). Reflections on doing training for the World Health Organisation's mental health gap action program intervention guide (mhGAP-IG). *International Journal of Mental Health, 48*(4), 309–322.

Musyimi, C. W., Mutiso, V. N., Nandoya, E. S., & Ndetei, D. M. (2016). Forming a joint dialogue among faith healers, traditional healers and formal health workers in mental health in a Kenyan setting: Towards common grounds. *Journal of Ethnobiology and Ethnomedicine, 12*(4), 1–8.

Okoroafor, S. C., & Christmals, C. D. (2023). Task shifting and task sharing implementation in Africa: A scoping review on rationale and scope. *Healthcare, 11*, 1200.

Olivier de Sardan, J.-P., Diarra, A., & Moha, M. (2017). Travelling models and the challenge of pragmatic contexts and practical norms: The case of maternal health. *Health Research Policy and Systems, 15*(Suppl 1), 60.

Patel, V., Flisher, A. J., & Cohen, A. (2012). Chapter 9: Global mental health. In M. H. Merson, R. E. Black, & A. J. Mills (Eds.), *Global Health: Diseases, programs, systems and policies* (3rd ed.). Jones and Bartlett.

Read, U. M. (2019). Rights as relationships: Collaborating with faith healers in community mental health in Ghana. *Culture, Medicine and Psychiatry, 43*, 613–635.

Ridde, V., & Olivier De Sardan, J.-P. (2022). The development world: Conflicts of interest at all levels. *International Review of the Study of Development, 249*, 247–269.

Simwaka, A., Peltzer, K., & Maluwa-Banda, D. (2007). Indigenous healing practices in Malawi. *Journal of Psychology in Africa, 17*(1), 155–162.

Solera-Deuchar, L., Mussa, M. I., Ali, S. A., Haji, H. J., & McGovern, P. (2020). Establishing views of traditional healers and biomedical practitioners on collaboration in mental health care in Zanzibar: A qualitative pilot study. *International Journal of Mental Health Systems, 14*(1), 1–10.

Sood, A. (2016). The global mental health movement and its impact on traditional healing in India: A case study of the Balaji temple in Rajasthan. *Transcultural Psychiatry, 53*(6), 766–782.

Steinforth, A. S. (2009). *Troubled minds: On the cultural construction of mental disorder and normality in southern Malawi*. Peter Lang.

Summerfield, D. (1999). A critique of seven assumptions behind psychological trauma Programmes in war-affected areas. *Social Science and Medicine, 48*(10), 1449–1462.

Summerfield, D. (2008). How scientifically valid is the knowledge base of global mental health? *British Medical Journal, 336*(7651), 992–994.

Summerfield, D., & Hume, F. (1992). War and posttraumatic stress disorder: The question of social context. *Journal of Nervous and Mental Disease, 181*, 522.

Summerfield, D., & Toser, L. (1991). Low intensity war and mental trauma in Nicaragua: A study in a rural community. *Medicine and War, 7*, 84–99.

Tobert, N. (2017). *Cultural perspectives on mental wellbeing*. Jessica Kingsley.

Udedi, M. (2016). *Improving access to mental health services in Malawi*. Ministry of Health Policy Brief. MoH.

Udedi, M., Swartz, L., Stewart, R. C., & Kauye, F. (2013). Health service utilization by patients with common mental disorder identified by the self-reporting questionnaire in a primary care setting in Zomba, Malawi: A descriptive study. *International Journal of Social Psychiatry, 60*(5), 454–461.

USGS. (2018). *Tsunami generation from the 2004 M=9.1 Sumatra-Andaman earthquake*. https://www.usgs.gov/centers/pcmsc/science/tsunami-generation-2004-m91-sumatra-andaman-earthquake

van Breugel, J. W. M. (2001). *Chewa traditional religion*. CLAIM.

Whitley, R. (2015). Global mental health: Concepts, conflicts and controversies. *Epidemiology and Psychiatric Sciences, 24*(4), 285–291.

Wickramage, K. (2006). Sri Lanka's post-tsunami psychosocial playground: Lessons for future psychosocial programming and interventions following disasters. *Intervention, 4*(2), 163–168.

Wright, J., & Jayawickrama, J. (2021). "We need other human beings in order to be human": Examining the indigenous philosophy of Umunthu and strengthening mental health interventions. *Culture, Medicine, and Psychiatry, 45*, 613–628.

Wright, J., & Maliwichi-Senganimalunje, L. (2020). Pluralism and practicality: Village health Workers' responses to contested meanings of mental illness in southern Malawi. *Anthropology & Medicine, 27*(1), 32–48.

CHAPTER 5

'Bringing It All Back Home'—Coloniality in the UK

5.1 Biomedicine as the Indigenous Healing System—Mental Health in the UK

> He began to wonder whether we could ever make psychology so absolute a science that each little spring of life would be revealed to us. As it was, we always misunderstood ourselves and rarely understood others. Experience was of no ethical value. It was merely the name men gave to their mistakes ... All that it really demonstrated was that our future would be the same as our past.
>
> Oscar Wilde. *The Picture of Dorian Gray*, 1891.
>
> Wilde (1992, p. 73)

Everyday discussion in contemporary UK, whether in conversation, in print, on screen or on social media, is increasingly peppered with the language of 'emotions' and 'mental health'. Concern for the impact of whatever event or experience (good or bad) on the feelings of the persons involved has become seen as significant and of public interest. It's as if the language of psychology and mental health has escaped the therapist's consulting room and unveiled a hegemony that advocates an individual's personal 'mental health' as exclusive to an understanding of them and as a sense of their identity. As we have discussed in Chap. 2, terms such as "stress", but also "anxiety", "depression", and "trauma" are no longer

J. Jayawickrama, J. Wright, *Under the Gaze of Global Mental Health*, The Politics of Mental Health and Illness,
https://doi.org/10.1007/978-3-031-78258-9_5

simply professional or clinical terms but have instead, through medicalisation, entered a public consciousness as anticipated and predictable reactions to certain life events or circumstances. The definition of 'mental health' in the UK Mental Health Act 1983 is an interesting example of the wholesale acceptability of an ill-defined concept. According to Part 1—Application of the Act, mental disorder means any disorder or disability of the mind. This is not a definition at all but is simply a tautology. However, when something is acknowledged as real, it becomes real in its values. Using extrapolations from survey material from the UK in 2007, one in four people experienced a mental health problem in the year 2007 (McManus et al., 2009). In 2014 it was estimated that every week one in six people were experiencing a health issue that might constitute a mental health problem (McManus et al., 2016). In simple mathematics, this means that there were about 20 million people in the UK suffering from mental health problems—a prevalence of disorder made 'acceptable' to the UK public through the successful adoption of a mental health hegemony. In this, it appears that the clinical category of, for instance, "depression" has evolved in the public mind to more generalised experiences of "distress", "despair", "sadness", "gloominess", and "pessimism", the respite for any of which will be treatment; usually through the prescription of anti-depressants (Wakefield & Horwitz, 2007; Summerfield, 2006). This, despite a meta-analysis of research on anti-depressants showing response levels that struggle to transcend the placebo effect (Kirsch et al., 2008).

It is within this backdrop, where notions of 'mental healthism' are occupying the social space and the neoliberal economic climate of austerity is resulting in cuts to mental health services and welfare systems, that the particular concept of 'mental health' within UK society and mental illness services need to be understood. It may seem peculiar to be comparing the UK with countries from the Global South in a discussion of colonialism and mental health, not least because, as we have seen, the Global North was the source of imperialism that fuelled the colonialism of the eighteenth and nineteenth centuries and globalisation in the late twentieth century. As such, knowledge and values from the Global North might quite naturally be seen as the basis for the dominant epistemology around mental health and illness in the UK. Indeed, one might say that Western psychiatry is its indigenous healing system, but is this so? It might seem counter-intuitive to apply the framework of colonialism to such mental health care and healing systems, and yet, on the contrary, such an analysis helps us to understand the very underpinnings and functioning of colonialism and its links to classism, which continue to divide British society.

5.2 The Coloniality of Biomedicine in the UK

In the UK, colonialism has been discussed as a concept of the past and as external to the country. The UK school system, for instance, rarely teaches the historical impacts of colonialism on the colonised, where the freedom of individuals on every continent was threatened. However, what is equally forgotten is how the British Empire was treating its own poor and disadvantaged. For through the seventeenth to nineteenth centuries' zenith of British imperialism, the accumulation of wealth benefitted just a very small elite of the population (Andrews, 2021). The material conditions and health of the majority poor was dire. Certainly, developments in water and sanitation, housing and education led the way to improvements in public health and later biomedical discoveries in germ theory, immunisation, and increased access to such innovations (especially to socialised health care systems like the National Health Service). Nevertheless, inequality remained a continuity, with those with most resources having access to greater opportunities for health through standards of living and private health care. Such inequalities mirror colonialism (Ferro, 1997) with its damage to the health of all sections of societies evident from Wilkinson and Pickett's (2010) research which reveals how the gaps between rich and poor within a society influences the health and wellbeing of all. Continuities of the poor's experience of illness (mental and physical) sustain the link between health and poverty in the UK—from Dickensian times to this day—not just from their experience, but from their representation, mirroring the colonisers' attitude to the colonised. With the British Empire benefitting such a small proportion of the population—the ruling elite—the imperial experience was largely a matter of 'class' (Porter, 2004; Anderson, 2006). In a study of the architecture of British colonialism Cannadine (2001) observed that British people of all classes shared a vision of British society as ordered, graded and hierarchical of race, class and gender. This image, Cannadine asserts, was the vision of the society that shaped an Empire constructed in the image of the home society. Seen in this light, the experiences of the colonised and colonisers both mirror social hierarchies and are mutually reinforcing through their structures and institutions.

For these ideas have created a hegemony of British ideals and white superiority that have become entrenched and repeated in dominant cultural narratives that have encompassed scandals to this day. The Grenfell Fire Disaster[1] (MacLeod, 2018) and the Windrush Scandal[2] (Slaven, 2021) are two recent examples of this type of narrative, and which on a wider scale appears to embolden powerful international corporate interests, environmental degradation and attitudes to climate impacts.[3] Within such a system, inequalities are rendered inevitable and lead to an acceptance of economic policies such as austerity, reductions in collective welfare, and identifying certain people as 'undesirable' (Heath, 2016). So, just as the poor in eighteenth-century England were blamed for being feckless, and ridiculed for their conditions, today in the UK, with its hegemony about individuals' 'mental health', the poor and disadvantaged are increasingly labelled as suffering from mental illnesses. In neither instance is the underlying problem of socio-economic deprivation questioned, and as Narayanaswamy (2024) reflects in her analysis of de-colonising contemporary 'development', "(neo)coloniality actually creates very similar types of divisions and outcomes in terms of 'haves' and 'have-nots' the world over" (p. 232). As Heath succinctly puts it, "Empire is no longer merely 'out there' in other parts of the globe. The disdain for human life that underpinned it has been brought home" (Heath, 2016).

According to Department for Work and Pensions (DWP) data in 2021/2022 around one in six people in the UK were in relative low income (relative poverty) before housing costs. This rises to just over one in five people once housing costs are accounted for. According to the Joseph Rowntree Foundation, four million British workers were living in poverty in 2019, a figure that had risen by over half a million compared

[1] The Grenfell Tower fire was a huge fire that broke out on 14 June 2017 in Grenfell Tower, a large block of flats in west London in the UK. In this fire, seventy-two people, predominantly from ethnic minority communities, died despite years of inaction by authorities over safety concerns of their high-rise residential tower block.

[2] The Windrush scandal was a British political scandal that began in 2018 concerning people who were wrongly detained, denied legal rights, threatened with deportation, and in at least 83 cases wrongly deported from the UK by the Home Office. Many of those affected had been born British subjects and had arrived in the UK before 1973, particularly from Caribbean countries, as members of the "Windrush generation" (so named after the Empire Windrush, the ship that brought one of the first groups of West Indian migrants to the UK in 1948).

[3] In these scandals, the British Government departments, local authorities and commercial organisations were found to have covered-up years of neglect and inaction.

with 2014 (Joseph Rowntree Foundation, 2019). According to McDaid et al. (2022), poverty and economic recession in the UK increased mental health problems among people, and mental health problems cost the UK economy at least £117.9 billion per year. Poverty can therefore be seen to be a significant contributor to people's experiences of distress in the UK, and these experiences are framed in a particular cultural tradition.

5.3 Coloniality and Inequality

Following the often protracted and bloody sacrifices of colonised peoples fighting for liberation, and when the imperialism of the Global North was no longer morally sustainable, the previously colonised territories took over their own governance. And yet despite such liberation, the previous colonial powers preserved the same trading power relations through global economic policies and agreements and 'neocolonialism' set in (Rodney, 1972; Andrews, 2021). This globalising drive has intensified over last four decades through organisations such as the World Bank and International Monetary Fund (IMF), as neoliberal global finance demanded competition, markets, privatisation, a reduced role for the state in health and welfare, and the promotion of the individual as 'consumer' across all continents, impacting the lives of people in the Global North as well as Global South. One universal consequence has been a burgeoning inequality between and within societies and accompanying increases in a wide range of health and social problems, from lower life expectancy and higher infant mortality to lowering educational attainment and increased homicide rates (Wilkinson & Pickett, 2010). Having established from earlier studies how inequality results in higher rates of mental illness and lower levels of child wellbeing, Wilkinson and Pickett (2018, p. xvii) turned their focus to how living in more unequal societies "changes how we think and feel and how we relate to each other". Their conclusions on the way inequality within a society and the drive for individualism creates a 'dislocation' in people's relationships mirrors Alexander's (2008) more concentrated focus on addiction which he saw as casualties from the breakdown of social cohesion and a disconnect from positive social relationships that are directly attributed to free market economic policies.

It's ironic then that despite the implication of inequalities and individualism to people's mental health, in 2007 the GMH movement launched its global mandate for 'mental health awareness' to be integrated into all aspects of health, social policy, health-delivery planning and the delivery of primary and secondary general health care (Lancet, 2007). Indeed, this intensification of the importance of 'mental health' coincided with the global financial crash of 2007 and economic downturn when the UK government made a clear policy decision to manage the economic deficit and recovery through austerity measures laid on the public purse—an intensification of neoliberal economic policy that had commenced in 1980s. Not surprisingly, while the lifestyles and life-chances of all but the very rich were affected, those with the least suffered most from the cuts in welfare, education, housing support and public services. Key markers of population health and wellbeing predictably declined as support for financial institutions and debt reduction rather than vulnerable populations were underwritten (Stuckler et al., 2017). And yet, at the very time when the collapse of social structures can be seen to be having the greatest threat to people's mental health and wellbeing, models like GMH emerged on the tailgate of public health successes in pandemics like HIV/AIDS, and despite its etiological and evidential limitations, offered an authoritative promotion of individualised 'mental health awareness' that had the effect of distracting from the social damage that measures such as austerity were causing. Far from promoting structural public health strategies and investment to alleviate distress, GMH offered a doubling down on mental illness as an individual threat to those weak and lacking in resilience. It was as if GMH was synchronous with neoliberal capitalist ideology (Moncrieff, 2008; Tseris, 2018).

Indeed, the promotion and perpetuation of this discourse by psychiatry can be seen in two ways. Firstly, despite significant evidential limitations outlined in Chap. 2, the focus on mental illness attributes people as having a chemical imbalance in the brain. Such individuation facilitates the neoliberal project (Moncrieff, 2008, p. 243). Secondly, the American Psychiatric Association's expansion of diagnoses in the DSM classifications of mental illness since 1980 has progressed an increasing focus on a person's ability to function, particularly in school and occupational environments, with diagnoses such as ADHD, autism, emotional dysregulation disorder, post-traumatic stress disorder, seasonal affective disorder, and defiant disorder. As Cohen (2018, p. 53) suggests,

> [B]iomedicine promises a range of corrections in line with neoliberal conduct, such as improved productivity and marketability as well as 'recovery' and the 'normalisation' of mental disorders for those who are at risk of deviating from their expected roles as workers, consumers, students, homemakers, and reproducers of the future workforce.
>
> Cohen (2018, p. 53).

Of course, this is not to say that people do not experience distress and suffer, only that it is how that distress is experienced and understood by the person and society which can be seen to have shifted. And this change aligns with the dominant discourse of neoliberal ideology and can in many ways be seen as a set of Western 'culture-bound' syndromes, since it denotes a (large) collection of signs and symptoms that is restricted to a culture by reason of certain psychosocial features (Stern et al., 2010). The emergence of neoliberalism in the 1980s led to significant socio-economic inequality among the global population. In health care, MacNaughton and Ahmed (2023) have argued that neoliberal ideology and policies intentionally block attempts at an equal distribution of health services. Instead, neoliberalism actively promotes a capital marketplace, which increases inequalities and prevents the practice of solidarity between the public and their health services by restructuring these services within an economic system that transfers the service obligations of governments to the private sector (MacNaughton & Frey, 2018). Within such systems, in the place of health promotion and disease prevention, which do not make profits, the private sector is incentivised to increase the labelling of populations as "unwell" or suffering from diseases, to enable the marketing of both pharmaceutical and non-pharmaceutical treatments and care.

In fact, to directly address the GMH claim of an exponential worldwide rise in the number of people suffering from mental health problems, which one might have thought would trigger a momentous call for structural political and socio-economic action and strengthening of communities, instead, what's offered is a targeted screening of individuals for mental illness and the promise of pharmacological or talking therapy. The accompanying promotion of mental health awareness and mental health 'literacy' further stoked the additional obligations on the 'responsible' citizen for self-surveillance and self-labelling (Cohen, 2018). However, the illuminating study by Amy Johnson described in Chap. 2 showed clearly how, outside disadvantaged and vulnerable groups affected by the financial crash, actual levels of distress within populations had not increased (Johnson, 2021). Instead, it is the way that mental health problems are understood and articulated that has changed fundamentally in line with the expanding hegemony. More and more people in the UK are seeking help, and these are disproportionately from poor and disadvantaged groups in society. As Korn (1997) has argued mental health experts such as psychiatrists, psychologists, and counsellors focus on the effects of external challenges on the mind, rather than the social, political, cultural, economic, and environmental roots of the difficulties since these issues are seen as beyond the scope of their practice. In the UK, there is always a close connection between poverty and mental health. Boardman et al. (2022) presents that poor people have higher rates of mental health problems, particularly severe conditions, than higher-income groups. According to Thomson et al. (2023), people who are living below the poverty line escalates the occurrence of common mental health conditions in the UK working-age adults by 2.5%, with an odds ratio of 1.21. In place of the demands for poverty alleviation and development solutions the public claim is for more financial resources for mental health care (Thomson et al., 2023; Boardman et al., 2015).

> Me and me bairn [child] are now struggling, because I lost my job. I am now on financial support and that is not enough. When I complained this to the job centre, they asked me to see me GP. Then the GP sent me to six sessions of counselling. Am I crazy to think that I need a job and look for a job? They just want to talk about how I feel, ... this is rubbish, ... ay.
>
> A young mother who lost her administration job at a university, Newcastle upon Tyne, personal discussion with one of the authors (March 2018).

Over the past 14 years of austerity, the UK has reduced mental health services to a bare minimum and the UK Parliament's Public Accounts Committee report (House of Commons Committee of Public Accounts, 2023) has exposed the resultant crisis in mental health care provision. An estimated 1.2 million people were on the waiting list for community mental health services and between 2016–2017 and 2021–2022 referrals to these services increased by 44%. Around 17,000 staff (12%) left the NHS mental health workforce in 2021–2022 and the staff vacancy rates in acute inpatient mental health services approximated 20% or more. As we have seen in earlier chapters, this mental health help-seeking is framed within the dominant hegemony, and whether individualised treatment or poverty reduction in the form of structural improvements are most effective is a separate argument. What is clear in this process of austerity is that while there is no attention towards structural improvements or investments to reduce poverty and inequality, even the individualised treatments that have themselves provided a cover for the neglect of structural change, are becoming still more scarce and unattainable for those in need. At the same time, in the face of these cutbacks in the formal mental health care system, the dominance of Western psychiatry has continued to expand into what has become known as the psy-professions in formal and informal health sector provision in the UK. This rise in the notion of 'mental healthism' advances the hegemony developed by psychiatry into the idea that mental health is everybody's concern (Mitchell et al., 2017) and that support and care is no longer reserved for the 'crazy'. What R.D. Laing described as "Psychophobia"—an intense fear of the mind—has been reimagined to place everyone in a persistent state of concern for our 'mental health' or 'sanism' that both privileges psychocentrism and preserves mental illness stigma (Fan et al., 2021; Ahrend, 2022). And thus, beneath the capitalist or neoliberal agenda, an uneasy alliance has been struck between psychiatry and other mental health professions, often with diametrically opposing views of medicalisation, to attend to people's individual distress and suffering. Within such a discourse, while psychiatry designates illness and treatment, and recovery philosophy retains the idea that mental illness is not something to be 'cured' but implies the need for personal growth, both nevertheless focus on individual change—which remains the requisite within the neoliberal capitalist agenda (Fig. 5.1).

Indeed, this widening of perceptions of mental health and mental illness contribute further to creating new markets for mental health itself, not just locally in Europe and North America, but globally. With individualism at its core, a person with a mental health problem, or the 'consumer', is asked to shop around for access to such provision. Although in the same way as some Western mental health care is available to elite urban Sri Lankans and Malawians, the affluent UK population may be able to afford private psychiatry or psychotherapy. But this is beyond the reach of the majority population who rely on an over-stretched and ever-decreasing NHS provision of mental health treatment and care. Such environments, which are over-represented in post-industrial areas of the UK such as in parts of the Northeast of England, Wales, and Scotland, have seen not just decades of a lack of financial and social investment, but also a sharp decline in state provision of health promotion and welfare. As we have seen, such inequalities create dislocations in communities that perpetuate distress and mental health problems and yet these are overlooked by those in power who are responsible for the neoliberal economic policies.

> Ay, I am terminally ill. I have a heart problem. One of the artilleries is very thin. Last week I was seriously ill, and my doctor said that if I continue to smoke, I don't have much longer to live. What's the point in giving up

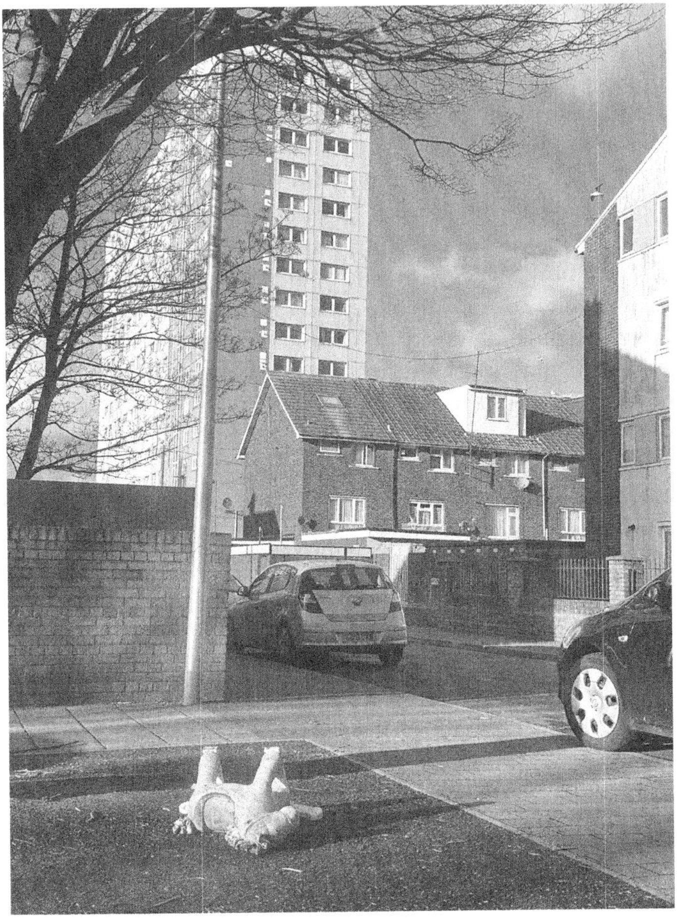

Fig. 5.1 Urban United Kingdom. (Photo: Sophie Wright, 2024)

smoking and living for another two or three years? I didn't smoke during my 17-year marriage and after she left me, I started smoking again. I don't have any interest in my family and not much of a social circle. I read quite a lot and play golf sometimes, but I am not really interested in any of these. Life is shit in this country and no one cares about others. My doctor diagnosed me as suffering from clinical depression. I took those anti-depressants for about one and half years. They make me pretty sick and do not allow me to be active. So, I quit taking them. I want someone to talk to, not some medication. But the doctor doesn't talk to me for more than five minutes. Various

therapists I have been to always analyse my childhood or want to change my behaviour. What is wrong with these people? Why can't they accept that this world is a shit place, and I don't enjoy it?
A taxi driver from Newcastle upon Tyne
Personal discussion with one of the authors (October 2009).

In his ethnography of community mental health teams (CMHT) in the UK, Moth (2018) identifies two examples of what he calls 'ethical professionalism' and resistance to managerialism among the CMHTs. In one, despite not within a formal contract of services they provide, the nurses facilitated a 'mental health matters' group with service users which sought to create an alternative space within which to "reframe user-practitioner power relationships and challenge 'the medical model... [and its] one size fits all' approach" (p. 148). Such an ethical commitment by the nurses and other CMHT members reflects a kind of resistance to the medically dominated hierarchy of the NHS and is undertaken under the gaze of neoliberal managerialism and the regular cost-containment and reorganisations of service provision. A second example Moth (2018) offers demonstrates even more explicit resistance in the face of service reduction. Here, the CMHT workers joined service users in a long campaign to lobby against closure and keep open a local 'drop-in' centre that had provided open access to support and demonstrates the CMHT workers' resistance to biomedical dominance and neoliberal reforms through the defence of wider "recovery-orientated and user-centred perspectives" (Moth, 2018, p. 149). Such resistance is all the more striking because usually, in the face of the demands on the UK mental health service systems and the precariousness of their jobs and roles, health workers 'survive' within organisations (by not even raise alarm when they are unable to meet demands of even rudimentary care. Instead, workers can find themselves as apologists or 'interpreters' like those seen in Malawi, where the dominant discourse of neoliberal reforms is not questioned. Where one might have expected a recognition that massive waiting lists and caseloads in community mental health teams would trigger an alert within the organisation that they were unable to fulfil their contracts to deliver safe and evidence-based interventions, instead, workers are encouraged to reduce their expectations, triage more intensively and add to waiting lists. The inadequacy and gaps in provision are reasoned as the result of the burden of mental illness which reinforces the need for psychiatry, rather than a more radical appraisal of the approach. Fearful of losing their job or influence, these 'interpreters' mask deficits and collude with the rationing of evidenced interventions. Like in Malawi, these 'interpreters' are genuine and well-meaning, but they are casualties of the precarious nature of services and the post-Fordist notion in neocapitalism where a perverse incentive exists in which the impression of work is more compelling than actual delivery and the continued myth of the adequacy of an individualised biomedical response to distress is maintained.

5.4 Understanding a Community's Distress—The Aberfan Disaster

As we have seen, as a post-industrial and increasingly secular society, in many ways the UK can be seen as embracing an understanding of mental health and mental illness that is culture specific (or even 'culture bound') and very attuned to the individualistic concept of personhood that is characteristic of Euro-American tradition (Jenkins & Barrett, 2004). The biomedical convention that posits the mind as focal and (in the case of illness) as defective, disintegrated, or dysfunctional in some way, creates the description, classification, and treatment of mental disorders. This centrality of the individual within illness is reflective of the self in neoliberal and consumerist contexts, and is reflected in contemporary notions of mental health or 'sanism' which dominate the discourses of people and their relationship to society. By their very nature, market orientated economics have reshaped the social and political contexts of people's experiences.

Yet, to what degree are these cultural values shared and to what degree might they be obscuring more traditional notions of collectivism and community? Might it be that these notions appeal to a dominant class or denote a dominant socio-political discourse—in a form of coloniality? It could be that the experience of crisis, whether that's ongoing poverty and deprivations or sudden shocks like the COVID-19 pandemic, summon a doubling-down on the demand for individual or personal protection and risk-reduction rather than a re-evaluation of the benefits and limitations of the individualistic endeavour.

The Aberfan disaster of 1966 represents a focal event in responses to disaster in the UK and came at a time when there was an expansion of psychiatric thought as modern, scientific, and worthy of popular debate. Its position in historical and socio-cultural context also came at a point when the significance of heavy industry to local and national prosperity was reserved, but at the same time neoliberal policies were beginning to plot a post-industrial future with the accompanying impacts on such communities. Significantly too, the disaster occurred at the cusp of a revolution in media communication and global exposure that shapes what are considered acceptable public, governmental, and international responses.

Aberfan in the Welsh hills was a traditional working-class community centred on coal mining. The richness of the coal seam had for generations created a level of wealth that had sustained the community, with all its associated commercial, social, and public services. Like so many villages in the Welsh coal fields, these services sustained a standard of living that, although often not far above a poverty level, nevertheless had a richness of community culture, including notions of work, gender roles and aspirations for subsequent generations. Not unusually in such established communities, this sense of culture imbibed in its members a value and confidence in collective endeavour and held a level of suspicion at outside authority.

When disaster struck on 21st October 1966 slippage from a coal tip led to a massive landslide. Within three minutes 144 people were dead, 116 of which were children at school. Few families escaped bereavement, and none escaped the impact. The experience of trauma and grief were immediate and total, and affected survivors, families, first responders from the emergency services, and members of the community who assisted in rescue attempts and the recovery.

Yet in the aftermath, despite intense media interest—with journalists and TV cameras positioned in Aberfan within hours of the disaster—there were no plans for any interagency or joined-up response from health and social services. Instead, members of the community took on the primary responsibilities and actively laboured in the recovery. Despite the many outside offers of support that was generated from the huge media expose, the local Aberfan services intervened sensitively—conscious of local opinion, suspicious of psychiatry and social work—and devised that only local GPs and one appointed social worker would be charged with supporting the traumatised community. The appointed social worker was even given time to gain the trust of the community as she began her work with the bereaved families. Community groups began to be formed and facilitated by locals, allowing people to talk through their experiences and emotions and to channel their anger (Johnes, 2002). Some groups—including singing groups—sprang up spontaneously as a way that men could find outlets for communal expression of their grief. While at this distance in time, it is easy to romanticise the responses of a community—for reactions are complex—the extent to which the community were able to suffer 'in private' and the fact that children returned to school in just over two weeks following the disaster appear to have been significant. This was speeded by the fact that at the time of the disaster an alternative school was already being constructed. Summerfield has noted these reactions as at odds with more recent disaster responses—where there is "an assumed vulnerability in a culture pre-occupied with trauma and emotional deficit" (Summerfield, 2005). Of course, there were undoubtedly psychological 'casualties', with up to half of a population of child survivors going on to experience symptoms that were later diagnosed as PTSD (Morgan et al., 2003). For a minority of survivors, the intensity of such experiences lasted long into adult life, although identifying which child was destined for long lasting distress was impossible to predict. Equally, experiences of anxiety and depression were no more elevated in the survivor population than in 'control' pupils, or in fact than those in communities of similar socio-economic environments (Morgan et al., 2003). So, for individuals it seems, resuming normal life within the family and community appears to have provided the most optimal chance of recovery.

Another aspect of recovery that seems key for communities as they emerge from a disaster is a collective form of healing. As we have seen, people within the Aberfan community experienced an intense feeling of trauma and loss. But they also experienced anger and guilt. The danger of the increasing size and precariousness of the coal tip had been identified several years prior to the disaster. These concerns had been ignored by authorities—the Merthyr Vale Colliery, the National Coal Board, and the government—and no action had been taken. The anger at the inaction of the authorities, together with a guilt that people might have argued more strenuously for change, were all understandable. But each was also underlain by the fundamental tension that the disaster resulted from the effects of the very industry that sustained the community and the loss of so many children impacted the community's very purpose of improving life for future generations.

> [T]he fact that mining was the main occupation of the area, meant that in many ways it had been a deprived community. It was made up largely of small old houses, and apart from the churches, chapels, and public houses, had had few amenities in the past. The loss of large numbers of young children in such an area seems especially tragic as they represented a better future.
>
> Lacey (1972, p. 258).

For a community to heal, and for individuals in that community to see meaning in their recovery, the social and political context of an event or disaster needs to be acknowledged by authorities. As Lacey further observed of the Aberfan experience "it seemed that real recovery only began to take place when this aggression started to subside" (Lacey, 1972, p. 258). It seems pertinent therefore to ask whether a focus on individual psychopathology—and the presumption of deficit—doesn't divert and inhibit discussion of the structural social and political factors and impact that are behind the disaster. In the case of Aberfan, a disaster inquiry was established and reported the same year of 1966, implicating the National Coal Board as responsible and concluding that the disaster could and should have been prevented. In the meantime, and in the years to come, the local authorities made considerable efforts NOT to psychopathologise the whole community. Whether such a response would be possible in our more contemporary UK society, with its ever-employed focus on individual trauma and recovery, and its lengthy public inquiries, is debateable. Radiven and Prideaux's (2021) analysis of the Grenfell Fire Disaster in 2017, found similar structural contexts being deflected by powerful interests and diverted by individualistic approaches to trauma. Both disasters demonstrate the way that communities were seen as dispensable, and profit was put before safety and human lives (Radiven & Prideaux, 2021). In this way, the adoption of the language and processes of biomedicine serves (perhaps unwittingly) to stifle the natural impulse of individuals and communities to understand the context of their shared experience. Similar to the exercise of power by a colonial authority, the control of the focus and meaning of an event extends a perspective of individual rather than collective loss and reduces the opportunities for empowerment. Indeed, it may therefore come as little surprise that, more than 50 years after the Aberfan disaster, disputes continue as to who is responsible for safeguarding communities surrounding the 2500 remaining disused coal tips in Wales (Morris, 2023).

5.5 Colonialism as the Exercise of Oppression, Division and Distress

From the perspective of a reader from the Global North this chapter encourages you to consider impacts of coloniality at home—and not always 'over there'. For readers from the Global South, it may have provided helpful context for your own experiences of being ruled or settled by powerful outsiders.

For, to turn the mirror of coloniality back onto the 'seat' of Empire and to expose its impacts is an example of what we described earlier as 'epistemic disobedience' and runs against accounts documented by the imperial power. But it is a disobedience that is gaining significant traction in examining the potential of the existing international governance systems and corporate interests to respond to the vast global challenges of poverty, inequality, social justice, environmental degradation and climate impacts. Justice should be at the centre of assessments of climate change impacts on health (van Daalen et al., 2023).

We have argued that the continuity of colonialism—of coloniality—in the UK provides a vital cultural framework for the continuance of a divided society and unequal class system which, as in Malawi and Sri Lanka, has changed the way we understand the experience of distress and suffering, and, just as crucially, the ways that societies endorse how to respond. This reshaping—largely from a collective to an individualistic understanding and response—is infused by ideas of capitalism. As we have seen in earlier chapters, global capitalism, as the ideology underpinning this coloniality, has become hegemonic in endorsing the biomedical responses even to social and political problems such as mental health and wellbeing. Indeed, the Césaire's 'boomerang effect' may well be a valuable lens through which to understand the origins and maintenance of racism in the UK's mental health services (Fernando, 2003).

For, as we have seen in this chapter, while people in the UK have benefitted significantly from free biomedical health services made universally accessible through the National Health Service, both biomedicine's evidenced limitations in the care of people with mental health problems and recent severe cuts and degradations of mental health and wider welfare and social services through government-imposed financial austerity measures have meant that the most vulnerable in society—the poor—become further underserved and disadvantaged. In response, we have seen how mental health professionals and people they are working with have adopted 'resistance' measures similar to those we have exposed in Malawi and Sri Lanka. And finally, as perhaps a portal to a previous world—prior to the establishment of globalised notions of mental health—the Aberfan disaster is offered as a reminder of the significance of a community's intrinsic—or indigenous—values. Here, Aberfan provides an example of a response not encumbered by globalised knowledges of mental health but that instead retained strengths of collective action and resolution rather than individualistic healing. It also underscores the importance that life events and experiences are not disconnected from their social and political context. In Aberfan, just as in Malawi and Sri Lanka, such context is critical to both social justice and healing. The following chapter will develop these themes of mobilising local indigenous understandings and resources into genuine and respectful collaborative approaches to the working with people and communities in distress.

References

Ahrend, E. E. (2022). *Sanity on the margins: A multidisciplinary literature review on Sanism*. Available at SSRN 4069055.

Alexander, B. K. (2008). *The globalisation of addiction: A study in poverty of the spirit*. Oxford University Press.

Anderson, B. (2006). *Imagined communities: Reflections on the origins and spread of nationalism* (revised ed.). Verso.

Andrews, K. (2021). *The new age of empire: How racism and colonialism still rule the world*. Allen Lane.

Boardman, J., Dogra, N., & Hindley, P. (2015). Mental health and poverty in the UK–time for change? *BJPsych international, 12*(2), 27–28.

Boardman, J., Killaspy, H., & Mezey, G. (2022). *Social inclusion and mental health*. Cambridge University Press.

Cannadine, D. (2001). *Ornamentalism: How the British saw their empire*. Oxford.

Cohen, B. M. Z. (2018). Marxist theory. In B. M. Z. Cohen (Ed.), *Routledge international handbook of critical mental health*. Routledge.

Fan, W., Qian, Y., & Jin, Y. (2021). Stigma, perceived discrimination, and mental health during China's COVID-19 outbreak: A mixed-methods investigation. *Journal of Health and Social Behavior, 62*(4), 562–581.

Fernando, S. (2003). *Cultural diversity, mental health and psychiatry: The struggle against racism*. Bruner-Routledge.

Ferro, M. (1997). *Colonization*. Routledge.

Heath, D. (2016, November 21). The ongoing effect of empire—In Britain. *The Conversation*. https://theconversation.com/the-ongoing-effect-of-empire-in-britain-67429

House of Commons Committee of Public Accounts. (2023). *Public accounts committee report: Progress in improving NHS mental health services*. UK Parliament.

Jenkins, J., & Barrett, R. J. (Eds.). (2004). *Schizophrenia, culture and subjectivity: The edge of experience*. Cambridge University Press.

Johnes, M. (2002). Aberfan and the management of trauma. *Disasters, 2000, 24*(1), 1–17.

Johnson, A. L. (2021). Changes in mental health and treatment, 1997–2017. *Journal of Health and Social Behavior, 62*(1), 53–68.

Joseph Rowntree Foundation. (2019). *UK Poverty 2018*. The JRF Analysis Unit. Joseph Rowntree Foundation.

Kirsch, I., Deacon, B., Huedo-Medina, T., Scoboria, A., Moore, T. J., & Johnson, B. T. (2008). Initial severity and anti-depressant benefits: A meta-analysis of data submitted to the Food and Drug Administration. *PLoS Medicine, 5*(2), e45.

Korn, L. (1997). *Community trauma and development*. University College, Dublin and the Center for World Indigenous Studies.

Lacey, G. N. (1972). Observations on Aberfan. *Journal of Psychosomatic Research, 16*, 257–260.

Lancet Global Mental Health Group. (2007). Scale up services for mental disorders: A call for action. *The Lancet, 370*, 1241–1252.

MacLeod, G. (2018). The Grenfell tower atrocity: Exposing urban worlds of inequality, injustice, and an impaired democracy. *City, 22*(4), 460–489.

MacNaughton, G., & Ahmed, A. K. (2023). Economic inequality and the right to health: On neoliberalism, corporatization, and Coloniality. *Health and Human Rights, 25*(2), 105–110.

MacNaughton, G., & Frey, D. F. (Eds.). (2018). *Economic and social rights in a neoliberal world*. Cambridge University Press.

McDaid, D., Park, A. L., Davidson, G., John, A., Knifton, L., McDaid, S., Morton, A., Thorpe, L., & Wilson, N. (2022). *The economic case for investing in the prevention of mental health conditions in the UK*. Mental Health Foundation.

McManus, S., Bebbington, P., Jenkins, R., & Brugha, T. (Eds.). (2016). *Mental health and wellbeing in England: Adult psychiatric morbidity survey 2014*. NHS Digital.

McManus, S., Meltzer, H., Brugha, T., Bebbington, P. E., & Jenkins, R. (2009). *Adult psychiatric morbidity in England: Results of a household survey*. Health and Social Care Information Centre.

Mitchell, A. J., Hardy, S., & Shiers, D. (2017). Parity of esteem: Addressing the inequalities between mental and physical healthcare. *BJPsych Advances, 23*(3), 196–205.

Moncrieff, J. (2008). Neoliberalism and psychiatry: A marriage of convenience. In C. I. Cohen & S. Timimi (Eds.), *Liberatory psychiatry: Philosophy, politics and mental health*. Cambridge University Press.

Morgan, L., Scourfield, J., Williams, D., Jasper, A., & Lewis, G. (2003). The Aberfan disaster: 33-year follow-up of survivors. *British Journal of Psychiatry, 182*(6), 532–536.

Morris, S. (2023, December 26). Wales fears another Aberfan as Westminster refuses to clean up tips, *The Guardian*. https://www.theguardian.com/uk-news/2023/dec/26/wales-fears-another-aberfan-as-westminster-refuses-to-clean-up-tips

Moth, R. (2018). 'The business end': Neoliberal policy reforms and biomedical residualism in frontline community mental health practice in England. *Competition & Change, 24*(2), 133–153.

Narayanaswamy, L. (2024). What is 'development' and can we 'decolonise' it? Some ontological and epistemological reflections. In H. Melber, U. Kothari, L. Camfield, & K. Biekart (Eds.), *Challenging global development. EADI global development series.*

Porter, B. (2004). *The absent-minded imperialists: Empire, society, and culture in Britain*. OUP.

Radiven, C., & Prideaux, S. (2021). Disasters in Aberfan and Grenfell. In C. Radiven & S. Prideaux (Eds.), *Crimes of states and powerful elites: A collection of case studies* (pp. 9–32). Anthem Press.

Rodney, W. (1972). *How Europe underdeveloped Africa*. Pambazuka Press.

Slaven, M. (2021). The Windrush scandal and the individualization of postcolonial immigration control in Britain. *Ethnic and Racial Studies, 45*(16), 49–71.

Stern, T. A., Fricchione, G. L., & Rosenbaum, J. F. (2010). *Massachusetts general hospital handbook of general hospital psychiatry-E-book*. Elsevier Health Sciences.

Stuckler, D., Reeves, A., Loopstra, R., Karanikolos, M., & McKee, M. (2017). Austerity and health: The impact in the UK and Europe. *European Journal of Public Health, 27*(4), 18–21.

Summerfield, D. (2005). Disaster mental health: Lessons from Aberfan. *BMJ, 330*, 254.

Summerfield, D. (2006). Depression: epidemic or pseudo-epidemic? *Journal of Royal Society of Medicine, 99*, 161–162.

Thomson, R. M., Kopasker, D., Leyland, A., Pearce, A., & Katikireddi, S. V. (2023). Effects of poverty on mental health in the UK working-age population: Causal analyses of the UK household longitudinal study. *International Journal of Epidemiology, 52*(2), 512–522.

Tseris, E. (2018). Biomedicine, neoliberalism and the pharmaceuticalisation of society. In B. M. Z. Cohen (Ed.), *Routledge international handbook of critical mental health*. Routledge.

van Daalen, K. R., Romanello, M., Gordon-Strachan, G., Peña, S. M. H., Cai, W., Tonne, C., & Lowe, R. (2023). Challenges in tracking climate, health, and justice over time and large geographical areas. *The Lancet Public Health, 8*(4), e255.

Wakefield, J., & Horwitz, A. (2007). *The loss of sadness: How psychiatry transformed Normal sorrow into depressive disorder*. Oxford University Press.

Wilde, O. (1992). *The picture of Dorian gray*. Wordsworth Classics.

Wilkinson, R. G., & Pickett, K. (2010). *The Spirit level: Why equality is better for everyone*. Penguin.

Wilkinson, R. G., & Pickett, K. (2018). *The inner level: How more equal societies reduce stress, restore sanity and improve everyone's well-being*. Penguin.

CHAPTER 6

Beyond Colonial Approaches

6.1 From Past to Future

This chapter builds on the ideas developed from Chaps. 3, 4, and 5 where the accounts from the different case examples reveal that ancient approaches survive as contemporary and relevant responses to distress, even in a globalised and increasingly connected world. From our examples from Malawi, Sri Lanka, and from the UK, we have shown how the traditional and biomedical worlds of healing are navigated within contemporary realities.

In Malawi, we have seen how the ancient philosophy of *Umunthu* underpins the way in which individuals and communities think about and deal with life problems, and as such becomes vital to understanding a person's distress and connecting to personal and communal healing. We also argued that when people are suffering from chronic poverty, and experiencing human-induced disasters such as famine, it is problematic just to focus on mental health and wellbeing. A farmer who has lost his harvest due to drought is of course distressed because he cannot feed and take care of his family. What support he requires needs to derive from his community networks and resources, including a development solution that seeks to actively resolve or provide contingency for his material losses. Such responses get closer to the real needs of the farmer than any biomedical mental health interventions.

J. Jayawickrama, J. Wright, *Under the Gaze of Global Mental Health*, The Politics of Mental Health and Illness,
https://doi.org/10.1007/978-3-031-78258-9_6

In Sri Lanka, we have seen how the use of the Hindu and Buddhist concepts of Karma help people to deal with distress (Radhakrishnan, 1950; Radhakrishnan, 1963). The experiences of a 30-year-old war, natural hazards such as tsunami, floods, and droughts, as well as the current political and economic crisis has been used to elucidate the very considerable community strengths. As in Malawi, people in Sri Lanka are being dominated by development approaches that are based on Euro-North American philosophies and ideas of development. After all the conflicts and disasters over the past 50 years, the entire Sri Lankan society may be described as distressed, and yet they have been shown to carve out effective and meaningful local responses to such tragedies. It is also a distress that can be channelled into the pursuit of social, political, and economic change. The 2022 protests by Sri Lankan citizens against the President and governments' catastrophic political, socio-economic and environmental policies since 1948 can be seen to have been a result of this distress. Over the past 75 years, the Sri Lankan society has tended to turn towards violence to resolve social, political, and economic problems. The 1958 riots, the 1971 youth uprising, the 30-year-old war, and many other incidents are examples of this. However, in 2022, the social discourse during the socio-economic hardships shifted and people turned away from violence to engage in a process of peaceful protests, which resulted in the President's resignation. Distress, within the current context, and in combination with previous experiences, helped ordinary Sri Lankans to peacefully change their government.

In the UK too, we have shown how, despite a culture rooted in post-enlightenment thinking rather than ancient philosophy, examples of collective identities, the acknowledgement of distress and infrastructural resources are key to support each other in examples such as the Aberfan disaster of 1966 (Eyre, 2019). The job losses, rising house bills, and severe economic recession has pushed many poor and marginalised populations into suffering through poverty. As in Malawi and Sri Lanka, support must encompass how the community can respond to the sources of distress, and not simply focus on its individual expressions.

Indeed, more recent evidence of communities' COVID-19 pandemic responses (Breen, 2021) confirms the importance of harnessing social support, and that although wellbeing for most people dipped during the pandemic, these bounced back after the end of lockdown restrictions. However, for the already underserved and vulnerable, the further isolation and disruption to relied-upon services have resulted in a widening of mental health inequalities (Di Gessa et al., 2022). Such evidence shows the significance of structural responses (both inside and outside of the health sector) to people's lives and experiences of distress. What we are arguing here is that essentially, given resources and opportunities, people can draw strengths from the political, social, economic, cultural, and environmental structures, even when they are 'falling apart'.

The key miscalculation of GMH is the medicalisation of mental health and wellbeing through its conversion of social suffering into mental suffering (Sinha, 2023). Even the way this is articulated in the Sustainable Development Goals produces a reductionist, economic, individualised and pathologised response to poverty (Mills, 2018). So, despite its promise to alleviate illness and suffering, its impact is frequently the opposite. Instead of improving health and wellbeing, an exclusive focus on 'symptoms' of mental illness ahead of people's functioning, especially where resources are limited, leads to overmedication, incarceration, and no reduction in mortality (Hengartner, 2017; White et al., 2017; Sinha & Ranganathan, 2020). The stigma of mental health problems too is not improved by GMH explanation and diagnosis. Percudani et al. (2004) found people's employability worsened and a study of caregivers in Malawi indicated increased concern and distance from the mentally ill person (Sefasi et al., 2008). In a systematic review, Angermeyer et al. (2011) showed that biomedical causal attributions for mental illness were associated with less tolerant attitudes and stronger rejection of people. In practice across the two case studies, and elsewhere in our research work, both authors have seen how well-meaning physicians have 'protected' patients from the societal stigma of a mental illness label by not informing the patient of their diagnoses, but still prescribing medication (Wright et al., 2020). So much for the value of the 'mental health literacy' element of GMH!

Just as important, as we have seen, such medicalising also displaces other systems of healing, such as the Ayurveda, Siddha, and Deshiya Chikitsa in the Indian sub-continent (Halliburton, 2023; Sood, 2016). People always draw their strengths from what they know. From organising and conducting a ritualistic sacrifice for dead ancestral gods to wish for successful harvest in Malawi to Hindu and Buddhist ceremonies to a wish for the wellbeing of people that are suffering in Sri Lanka to prayer sessions in a Christian church in Gateshead in the UK are some of these strategies. Regardless of the country, people, especially when they are suffering, come together to help each other. Sharing whatever little harvest in Malawi; organising relief for disaster-affected people in Sri Lanka; and foodbanks in the UK are some examples. These are not just places to bring practical solutions, but also gatherings to share distress—feelings, emotions, and experiences—with each other. This is the people's ability to think in a non-linear fashion.

6.2 Beyond Linear Thinking

The following example was told by a Rwandan refugee living in Lilongwe in Malawi in 2006 (Jayawickrama, 2010, pp. 154–156). We offer this account, not to exhibit the litany of loss, abuse, and crisis that an individual has faced, (although certainly we acknowledge that this is a harrowing and distressing account to read) and certainly not to compare this person's experiences with the losses, abuses and trauma felt by any other persons. But rather to illustrate how a person's personal, historical, and social context positions their own understanding of distress and its resolution.

> Caroline is from Rwanda. Her parents were from two different tribes – her father was a Hutu, and her mother was a Tutsi. They were a happy family, and her parents loved each other very much. Her father was a businessman, and they had enough money to provide a good life for their four daughters. In 1994 the violence started, and a group of people came into her house. Caroline's parents and three sisters were killed. However, a member of the gang didn't want to kill Caroline; he wanted to marry her. She was unsure what this was but agreed to marry this man who had taken a part in killing her family. After a while they had a daughter and lived a life together.
>
> However, Caroline's maternal uncle didn't like the fact that she had survived. He wanted to claim her father's entire property for himself. As her uncle was a powerful man within the tribal system, he managed to kill her father in-law and imprisoned her brother-in-law. Caroline's husband ran away without knowing that she was pregnant again. Caroline continued to visit her brother in-law in the prison, as he was the only relative who had been kind to her. Her mother in-law kept accusing her of bringing bad luck to the family. Because of these unbearable accusations, Caroline somehow found a way to help her brother in-law escape from prison. The day he escaped, her uncle came with the police and arrested her. The police tortured her – they burnt her chest and beat her head till she bled. After pleading to her uncle, they released her on the basis of her daughter's welfare. But Caroline's friend, who was married to another powerful man in the system, managed to inform her that they were going to kill Caroline and her daughter. The friend helped Caroline escape to Tanzania in 2002. Caroline gave birth to a baby boy on her way to Tanzania.

In Tanzania Caroline and her children were treated very badly because of their mixed ethnicities. Her wounds from the torture were still present and she suffered a lot. Somehow, Caroline managed to find her husband; however, he did not want to see them. He used to beat her and the children. One day he beat her up so badly she ended up in hospital. One day he came to the hospital to give her two choices: one was to go to Rwanda where her uncle could kill her; the second was to live in Tanzania, but that he was planning to leave. Caroline asked him why he had saved her on that first meeting. He could only apologise to her and explained that he could not deal with her mixed ethnicity. He elaborated, saying that Caroline's uncle had found out that she was with him again and had threatened to kill his mother if he helped her. After much pleading from Caroline and further beatings from him, he brought them to Malawi in early 2004.

When they arrived in Malawi, Rwandan refugee communities became suspicious about Caroline. They thought she was spying for her uncle, who was now a very powerful man in the Kagame government in Rwanda. This led her husband to move them from the refugee camp to a house in Lilongwe city. He did not allow her to leave the house and her suffering continued. After some time, Caroline's husband changed a bit – he found a better house and started a small business. They had a good standard of life and Caroline realised she was pregnant again. This was the time she heard from a neighbour that her husband was having an affair with another woman. He stopped caring about Caroline and the children – he didn't bring any food to the house and sometimes did not come home for days. Caroline thought if they were to survive, she must develop friendships with the local community and learn the language. However, as gratitude for saving her, she continued to care for her husband.

One night Caroline gave birth, alone, in the house. Everything went well and her husband came later to take her to the hospital. After she came back from the hospital her husband left her again. He did not come home for months. Caroline and her children were supported by the friends she found in the local community. One night she came out from the house to go to the toilet. There were two men outside. They took her back into the house and raped her. The rape and beatings lasted for hours. After the men left, her eldest daughter went to help Caroline. She was on the floor, covered in blood and unable to move. Her daughter kept asking her what had happened and wanted Caroline to laugh with her so she could confirm that Caroline was alive. After about 30 minutes Caroline's husband came back. He refused to believe she had been raped and accused her of having affairs with other men. He told her that he did not want to be with her anymore and left the house. She has never seen him again. Next day Caroline went to the police to make an official statement about her rape, this would also enable her to go to the hospital. In the hospital they treated her and tested her for HIV/AIDS. Caroline was negative. After three months they tested her again and she was still negative.

She started her life with her children again. Her friends in the Malawian community are helping her and she has heard that her husband left Malawi in 2006 with his second wife. Caroline is struggling with no job or plans for future. However, she does odd jobs to keep her family going and tries to be positive about the future. Caroline thinks it is a worthwhile struggle. One day she will find good educational opportunities for her children, and they will live a good life. She is not worried about her husband or what has happened. Caroline thinks that it is God's will that she has to suffer and is happy to accept this. She thinks that towards the end of this dark tunnel of suffering, she will find the light of satisfaction and happiness. She finds that she is now much happier than she was with her husband and enjoys her time with her children, but she spends sleepless nights and worries about the following problems:

- Fear for the security of her children as the Rwandan refugee communities are angry with her as they think that she is a spy for her uncle.
- Because of this security problem Caroline cannot leave her children at home so as to get a job.
- Caroline wants to find asylum in a country where there are no Rwandan communities.
- Worry about her children's education and future.
- Finding help for her present and future problems. She finds it very difficult to deal with all the agencies she meets that want to discuss her feelings about her past.
Jayawickrama (2010, pp. 154–156).

Like Caroline, people do not separate and dissect their life story from problems and challenges. No matter how stressful, scary, and catastrophic, people have their ways to draw strength through their political, socio-economic, cultural, and environmental context. This is people's personal knowledge and must be respected. Unfortunately, as we have seen in previous chapters, the linear scientific analysis of an individual's internal world that is privileged in the biomedical mental health framework provides a deficit model that fails to grasp the realities of people's complex lived experiences, including their strengths.

When people don't share an understanding of the medicalised or biomedical mental health concepts or they are not plausible to their experience, it is not a surprise that people respond in different ways. We have seen this reaction as people seek help and treatment elsewhere, sometimes concurrently with biomedicine, while even the health workers employed within the biomedical system can be found to adapt their advice and interventions to be more plausible to both them and their patients (Wright & Maliwichi-Senganimalunje, 2020). As we have seen, this represents a 'resistance' to a dominant espoused ideology, without which, people are stuck in a kind of structural oppression, which does not allow them to overcome their distress. The following example from the UK shows this structural oppression, veiled as it is by biomedicine's assumed beneficence, and there are many similar examples in Malawi, and Sri Lanka:

> In her late 30's Georgia fell in love with an immigrant from Rwanda. Because of this, her Christian and English family decided to kick her out of their home. After two years of marriage, the couple had a beautiful daughter. The same year she was born, Georgia's husband had to leave the UK due to immigration issues. Georgia was then alone with a new-born daughter and without any family support. However, with the little help she received from her neighbours, Georgia managed to find babysitting for her daughter, so she could find work in the nearby hotel. Years went by, and Georgia's daughter started to go to school. Since the first day, her school and classmates had the problem to figure out whether she is a black child or white child. Many of her classmates did not want to be friends with her. Georgia was furious and she changed the school. In new school, Georgia received complaints from teachers that her daughter is aggressive, unruly, and disobedient. She tried to explain her background and situation to teachers, but Georgia and her daughter were referred to the social services. They took them to a psychiatrist and even without talking to them, he diagnosed Georgia's daughter as suffering from attention deficit hyperactivity disorder (ADHD) and immediately put her on medication. The girl who was once active, creative, and imaginative at school and at home, is now very quiet, silent, and sleeps a lot. Since starting medication, she also began to eat excessively and put on a lot of weight. Georgia is very upset, sad, and distressed about her daughter's situation without knowing what else to do. The school, on the other hand, reported to Georgia that her daughter is now peaceful, orderly, and obedient!
>
> A single mother from York
>
> Personal discussion with one of the authors (March 2022)

This is just an example how the biomedical mental health interventions are used to identify dis-ease and obtain an outcome without any appreciation of the person's socio-cultural context or particular lived experience. As we described previously, this is the same kind of "development oppression" for which the MGMH has become a vehicle.

In aspiration too, the implementation of intensive MGMH interventions such as through the Treatment Gap programme (WHO, 2008, 2010) is not either affordable or practical at a population scale in low- and many middle-resource settings (Sinha, 2023). Indeed, even in austerity-strapped high-income countries, the reductions in mental health care provisions reflect a similar inability to eradicate the 'treatment gap' (Sashidharan et al., 2016). For GMH has an overreliance on psychotropic medication (White & Sashidharan, 2014), fails to respond reflexively to local environments (Kirmayer & Pedersen, 2014) and its very method of design is open to question (Mills & Hilberg, 2019). In a fascinating but rare example of research into the perspectives of workers from the Global South who were in receipt of GMH frameworks rooted in the Global North, Taylor and Burgess (2019) reported workers' impressions that suggested Western psychology had a limited role, needed to account for unique cultural worldviews and practices and needed to address the power imbalances that were integral to the knowledge exchange.

Of course, such notions bring to the fore issues of power which get to the heart of the colonial approach that we have articulated throughout this book. As we have seen from our case examples, most often these exertions of power derive from outsiders (usually Western countries and Western-based organisations), and we have described these as colonial enterprises. But power and influence are also exerted when institutions, professions, and organisations from within a country exercise power and influence over local indigenous communities or groups. We have previously linked such actions to the influence of local 'interpreters' of colonial thinking (Wright & Jayawickrama, 2021), and similar exercises of power are seen in the actions of elite or professional classes within higher resource countries like the UK.

Within a broad critique of the conduct of a significant element of development aid, Ridde and Olivier de Sardan (2022) draw particular attention to the inadequacy of introducing standardised interventions beyond their original contexts. 'Travelling models' as they term them are reproduced in diverse settings in almost identical formats and fail to offer more than rhetorical acknowledgement of cultural and social norms which are critical to auguring sustainable improved health care. More culturally attuned interventions would encompass an appreciation of social norms of "modesty, decorum, mutual aid, collective action, gender relations, patron-client relations, education, the supernatural, death, relationships with the state" (Ridde & Olivier de Sardan, 2022, p. 79). With a similar emphasis Perera et al. (2020) have urged investment in meaningful adaptation within any exchange of knowledge between contexts that involves an analysis and shared reckoning of helping contexts. The same concerns are highlighted in Memon et al.'s (2021) challenge to those engaged in implementation research across cultures.

Even more unrecognised however, according to Olivier de Sardan et al. (2017, p. 80), is attention to the 'practice norms' of the health professionals and workers charged with delivering such interventions. Their real-life experiences include departures from learned professional practices (from which models are based) to certain alterations, adaptations, or "tricks" employed to accomplish the practice demands in their local context. Both these official and practical norms need to be addressed to bring about effective and sustained change (Olivier de Sardan et al., 2017).

Of course, the problem here throughout is the repeated one-way flow of knowledge (Lund, 2017). The paradox is that while globalisation can be defined as communication (of goods, services, and knowledge) which can bring promising external ideas, or ways of working, (including biomedical approaches), the actual exchange within a neoliberal capitalist global climate is overwhelmingly in one direction and is controlled by the powerful economies (Fricker, 2007). As a result, where the opportunities for learning of indigenous knowledge and healing systems may be present, these are most frequently ignored or dismissed as the innovations from Western countries dominate (Cox & Webb, 2015).

6.3 Emerging Alternative Approaches

And yet, an alternative does exist. By adopting a truly collaborative approach, so that the 'local' becomes sovereign and any innovations reflect the experiences and understandings of distress from that particular place and time. Somewhat sceptical of the overarching politics of international aid networks and processes, including a subverted evaluation mechanism, Ridde and Olivier de Sardan (2022), for instance, suggest actors instead need to focus on the 'practical norms' highlighted earlier. Which practice can be amended, modified, improved, or enhanced? Which must be abandoned? And how? And to the benefit of who? Asking such questions facilitates the development of 'tailor-made' rather than standardised approaches and considers the daily reality of social norms and practical norms. Of course, this is a more complicated, and yet potentially more promising, direction for any implementation or scale-up of mental health responses. Sustainability needs to be at the core of its mission by favouring, in short, the growth and development of local forms of support that prioritise social inclusion and long-term mental health recovery (Bayetti et al., 2023).

Indeed, with the impetus of critical scholars, researchers and engaged clinicians who are working with affected communities (e.g., White et al., 2017; Mills & Fernando, 2014; Fernando, 2014; Campbell & Burgess, 2012), there are signs that things may be moving in this direction. As Bayetti et al. (2023, p. 5) eloquently summarise:

> While some GMH advocates contend the economic constraints of LMICs (low- and middle-income countries) and the 'urgency' of the 'treatment gap' support market-driven 'values,' we suggest that this position may be short-sighted. We argue that mental health services in LMICs should be evaluated on more than their effectiveness in reducing symptoms and returning individuals to economic productivity.

Dispensing with a sole or even primary focus on biomedical approaches, Mathias et al. (2019) talk practically in their targeting of efforts to understand for whom does the intervention work, (or not), how does it work (or not work)? And in what context does it work (or not work)? Such a focus mirrors the resolute mission of the Butterfly Peace Garden described in Chap. 3, which asks the primary question, "is this in the best interests of the children?" (Butterfly Peace Garden, 2000, p. 1). In this way the central 'development' edict that those affected are most likely to determine acceptable and effective solutions echo theories of Wignaraja (1991) and Sen (1999). From their empirical work across continents Burgess and Mathias (2017) have developed a 'mental health competency' framework which encourages a focus on local engagement with communities in areas of formal and informal health provision.

Since current GMH solutions fail to address social determinants that maintain or impede mental wellbeing, Burgess et al. (2019) argue the need to move beyond adapting and 'scaling up' individual 'patient' interventions towards more clearly defining and operationalising 'social' approaches that impact structural conditions. Indeed, even one of the key early pioneers of GMH intervention approach, Crick Lund, is now turning attention to the complexities and challenge of targeting social determinants of mental health (Lund, 2023). As a behavioural scientist, Lund has begun to outline the challenges and advocate for building theoretical models that will inform programme/mid-range theory that explicitly attaches desired outcomes to human capability theory by Amartya Sen (1999). However, it is important to note that development is a question and challenge for many countries, including Malawi, Sri Lanka, and the UK. Coupled with colonial approaches, the mainstream development theories, policies, and practices are currently driven by the Bretton Woods Institutions, which were originally created to rebuild the war-ravaged Europe. The World Bank as we know it today had the original name of the Bank for Reconstruction and Development. The neoliberal policies implemented by both the International Monetary Fund (IMF) and World Bank have been responsible for much of the socio-economic crises we see in the contemporary world, and the inadequacy of the mainstream development paradigm based on linear and narrow economics and technocratic approaches has been recognised by many critiques (Wignaraja, 1991; Friedman, 2003; Prashad, 2014). As Friedman (2003) has argued, the capital marketplace has created competition at every level, which has had a miserable impact on everything from education to health to moral standards. Such critique argues that the time has come to move into nonlinear economics and development with a better framework to open the space for society with humanity as its foundation. Indeed, in the face of such deep-rooted political and socio-economic challenges, Oehring and Gunasekera (2024) argue the need to first establish an ethical component to promoting global health, one built on valuing the wellbeing of the disadvantaged, before any technical solutions are offered.

For, as our case studies have shown, there are alternative ways of understanding and responding to these challenges and human reactions. Sri Lankan traditional medicine (*Deshiya Chikitsa*) is based on Buddhist philosophy, and the ancient healers held wisdom about the mind-body balance for healthy living. The Dhammapada explains that greed and self-indulgence are the worst among all illnesses, and attachment creates the utmost sorrow (Radhakrishnan, 1950, Verse 203, p. 126). The Bhagavad Gita, a prominent Hindu text, points out that the passage to total freedom from suffering is not for the human that is indulging in too much food or eating too little, oversleeping, or sleeping less (Radhakrishnan, 1963). Moderation of everything we do has been an ancient principle in most traditions in Asia, Africa, Americas, and the Middle East. Explaining a model of development in the Ramayanam, Nandakumar (1971) recounts the great Tamil poet Kambar describing Ram Rajya, (a good society) where everyone had enough, and no one had more than enough. The ancient philosophies of *Umunthu*, Hindu, Buddhist, and Pagan traditions express an understanding of nature that advocates ways to adjust people's physical, mental, and spiritual processes. So, when knowledge is no longer seen as the exclusive preserve of outsider experts, extolling particular ideologies about the individual and its 'market-self', both old and new knowledge can materialise that is far more likely to have "credibility" (Patel, 2014) and represent a "plausible mechanism" (Lund, 2023). In this way Burgess and Mathias' (2017) framework commends the value of creating partnerships and 'safe social spaces' in which dialogue and critical thinking about people and their 'mental health' can be created in communities (p. 224). From India, Srinivasan et al. (2023) describe how NGOs are addressing care gaps through novel approaches that emphasise locally determined social recovery and inclusion—with common strategies for engaging communities, prioritising beneficiaries, co-opting resources, devolving care, re-organising communication, and recovery—in a way that reframes mental health as a development issue.

6.4 The Sovereignty of Place

Since peoples' perceptions and experiences are inseparable from their cultural meanings and practices, the importance of place, both geographically and cognitively, is critical for an understanding of distress, wellbeing, resilience, and hope. As we have seen throughout this book, experiences of distress are embedded in social life and the significance of the contexts to both the causes and the resolution of distress, reinforce the need for such plurality to be embraced. This might include traditional medicine and healing, spiritual, religious, as well as biomedical notions of health and health care. Indeed, only through an appreciation of such wider considerations can the opportunity for structural responses—social systems, infrastructure, and relational experiences—be realised to involve actively challenging environments and systems that perpetuate peoples' distress.

Allied to this notion of sovereignty of place is the importance of 'connection'—of a connection to place—where the experience of the external environment co-exists with a person's 'internal' experience, of thoughts and feelings, and of a 'spiritual' or metaphysical existence. Both biomedicine and some other forms of healing or medicine focus on the person's 'inner world' and describe the difficulties and challenges. Of course, biomedicine locates the problem here, and cognitive approaches seek to challenge the cognitions that are troubling or unhelpful to a person's wellbeing. However, for many peoples, the connection of themselves with their environment and place in the world extend far more broadly and deeply. In the UK, we have seen that many people might aim to retire to their hometowns, which is a hope for peace and tranquillity. Some will have particular relationships with their environments that span generations and may include ancestral legacies that traverse spiritual understandings. For example, both in Malawi and in Sri Lanka, people in traditional lands consider earth to be sacred. Losing land would have serious mental and spiritual impacts. Such conceptions expand biomedical understandings of ideas such as health and wellbeing—often with an intimate relationship with their ecosystems and accommodate experiences where people might be in direct contact with ancestral spirits. When people lose their lands, environments, and familiar surroundings due to "development" projects or poverty, there are consequences, which can be manifested as distress. Here people's experiences may not be seen as individual struggles, but as related to wider community or ecological distress. As we have explained in Chaps. 2 and 3, the rise of the discourse of mental health and illness as a major reason for suffering in the Euro-North American culture is an aspect of the medicalisation of life. However, people's experiences cannot be reduced to labels of mental health or distress. How can a mother's pride of the death of son fighting for the country in Sri Lanka be simply labelled as trauma? Or a couple in Malawi's sadness of the death of their infant baby due to poverty be labelled as depression? Or a young man in the UK who loses his job and then his girlfriend and chooses to no longer leave his apartment be diagnosed with simply an anxiety disorder? It's not that these biomedical diagnoses are not 'accurate' according to psychiatric traditions, but they offer only a fractional insight into people's problems. As the El Salvadorian philosopher Ignacio Martín-Baró argues, social catastrophes such as conflicts, disasters, and uneven development crises are not individual suffering but social suffering. Therefore, the treatment must be social, not individual (Martín-Baró, 1989, 1990). What we argue is that the "treatment" in most of these crises must be development rather than biomedically oriented. As Korn (1997) sees it,

> [T]he antidote to traumatic stress [or distress] is to take control – control of land, resources, political and economic structures.
> Korn (1997, p. 9).

Of course, even within this idea of 'sovereignty of place', there are inherent dangers of 'essentialising' certain peoples with assumptions about their understandings and experiences. As we have discussed, colonialism and globalisation—particularly in the form of global communication—have without doubt increased the coverage of ideas of mental health and wellbeing. Such exchange of ideas reduces the distinctness of cultural boundaries and creates more variegated and blended cultural trends. Many see this as accelerating rather than initiating a familiar acculturation phenomenon whereby cultures are 'fluid' rather than fixed and are instead made up of "a complex interaction of threads and patterns of behaviour, values and senses of self and identity" (Wolfe & Vitebsky, 2003 p. 66) which themselves become absorbed, contested, or develop new incarnations within cultures. It is in this way that ancient wisdom and traditions are sustained, developed or, (as we have seen, e.g., in Chap. 3, in the interaction of organised Christian or Islamic religions with Traditional African religion) become superimposed.

6.5 Collaboration with Humility

In Chap. 1 we introduced the idea of practising an 'epistemic disobedience' (Mignolo, 2009) in our approach to the complex challenges of intercultural exchanges. Such complexity in patterns of discourse and development which are present in all cultures' appeals for any 'outsider' to tread carefully in making assumptions about local understandings and practices.

Our collaborations over many years with people and communities experiencing different challenges of emergency, disaster, conflict, and uneven development settings as well as health challenges, have noted a series of values and behaviours that are visible in the most effective insider and outsider partnerships (Fig. 6.1). As explained in Chap. 1, we both as co-authors of this book practised and are practising this framework in our own collaboration. In that, we bring trust, collegiality, humility, equal participation, genuine engagement, and ownership and responsibility into this collaboration. This is truly a friendship that we can both be ourselves, learn from each other, and correct ourselves without being penalised. We

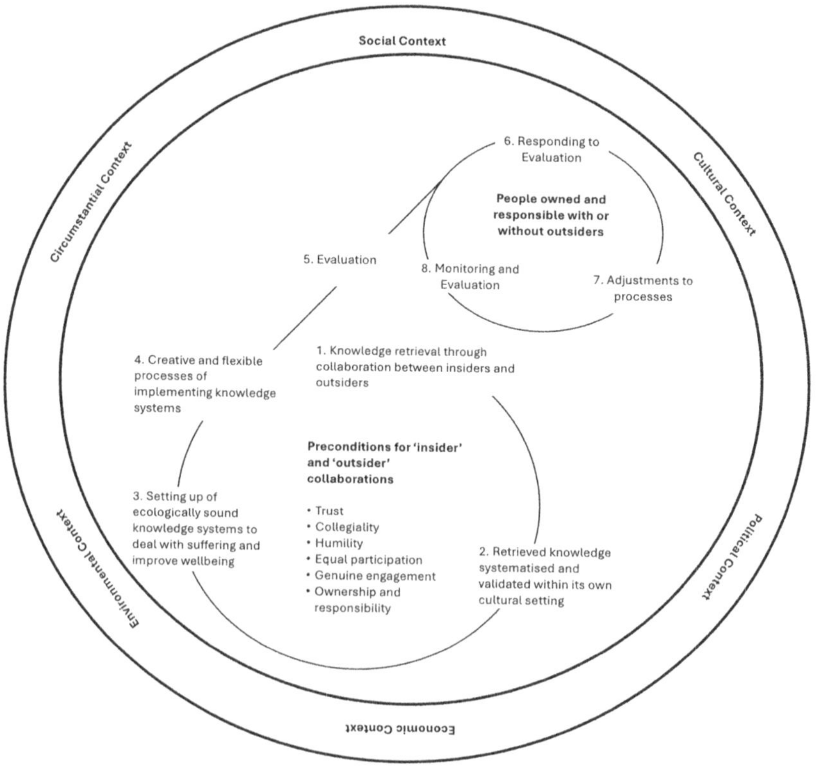

Fig. 6.1 Framework for "Insider" and "Outsider" Collaborations. (Adapted from Jayawickrama (2010))

both understand that we have certain experiences and knowledge, but we do not treat one experience and knowledge as better than the other. Through this approach, we collaborate as equal partners for change and to find new ideas. We both are outsiders to each other's worlds, while insiders of our own worlds.

For researchers or institutions from different contexts to collaborate through this framework, a shift in approach is required at both macro and micro levels. As we have discussed previously, the idea that an 'outsider' (usually, though not exclusively from the Global North) holds unique and critical knowledge that can be unquestioningly employed in new environments is no longer defensible. The North's assumed dominance and colonial continuities have received a sound theoretical and moral critique. Its exaggerated benefits have been seen across the globe as, even in disaster or emergency situations, it is local people that respond first to the call for assistance, and who are left to sustain the support long after any 'outsiders' depart. Likewise, poor populations in uneven development environments are frequently left to adjust again as projects 'complete' or are abandoned or indeed when a permanent 'internationalised presence' is established, as in the case of eye movement desensitisation and reprocessing therapy (EMDR) services in Cambodia (Jordan et al., 2022) or task-shifting interventions disrupt the shared consciousness of volunteers in India (Kottai & Ranganathan, 2020). A new approach must break from such dependence and disruption. At macro level then—as collaborations are designed and agreed—this needs to be with peoples most connected and affected. This will involve a break from traditional or formal aid partnerships where professional or institutional collaborations recreate colonial relationships, and often-siloed responses, to what are complex multisystem challenges. Instead, such new collaborations entail multiple partnerships, with multifaceted inclusive mechanisms that place the key decisions in the hands of local people (Heap et al., 2022).

Of course, in contrast to traditional aid relationships where donors retain and exercise decisive power, these are messier, less easily 'managed' and make for more complex lines of communication. And yet, while perhaps less attractive to donors looking for direct impact and accountability chains, its significant benefit derives from its effectiveness in connecting with those most affected, and through this a more fully realised provision of both ownership and choice in peoples' beliefs and aspirations for health and wellbeing (Nussbaum, 2011). Indeed, this fundamental break from traditional ways of funding, managing, and monitoring 'aid' from North to South mirrors the parallel call to decolonise research structures (Oti & Ncayiyana, 2021). It involves a calling out of oppressive engagements through the enactment of collaborative principles. If decolonisation is a radical reversal of power and influence—south to north—then giving voice to peoples most connected and affected through these collaborative principles is the only way to achieve this.

And so, these collaborations need to be extended at micro level too where the same values and behaviour (Fig. 6.1) underpin in the relationship created between partners:

1. Trust: Trust is a valuable element, which can only be built between two parties or two individuals. Building trust takes time, and energy to learn from each other. Sometimes, there are barriers such as language, cultural nuances, and unfamiliarity of the environment. Trust is a process that needs patience from both parties. Some of the requirements for trust comes through transparency, and accountability. Transparency comes through keeping honest about positive and negative aspects of the process. That can happen through accountability—being accountable for the understandings, actions, and outcomes.
2. Collegiality: In this process, collegiality means the actions, customs, and procedures agreed by both parties. This is also part of the trust building process. Not everything is correct or incorrect in both parties. Agreeing upon what works for both parties must come from honest, transparent, and accountable discourse. After agreeing, both parties seek to uphold those standards, procedures, and actions.
3. Humility: Understanding that one does not know is the foundation of humility. Realisation of one's ignorance and seeking answers comes through humility. In this process, both parties must learn from each other, which has to be practised through humility. Humility is also about thinking yourself less, but not thinking less of yourself. It is also the ability to relinquish pride, and yet still retain your dignity.
4. Equal participation: Based on trust, collegiality, and humility, both the parties can establish equal participation in the process. Equality comes through inclusion of ideas, thoughts, and also differences. Inclusion is also about respecting the differences of ideas, thoughts, and actions. This can only happen when there is humility and collegiality in both parties.
5. Genuine engagement: Through equal participation comes genuine engagement. Being genuine is also connected to transparency and accountability. Also, when both parties practise humility and collegiality through their trust for each other, it is easier to engage genuinely.
6. Ownership and responsibility: When there is genuine engagement, there is an ownership and responsibility of the process. When there is ownership and responsibility, that facilitates commitment and wanting to push for positive outcomes.

Our experience in different cultural contexts and from the accounts of insider and outsider partnerships indicate that those underpinned by such values and behaviours can create an environment for true learning and development. Through humility and respect for equal participation particularly, partners are able to share their experiences so that the boundaries between cultures are seen less as fixed positions from which essentialising and binary determinations are created, and more as "a complex interaction of threads and patterns of behaviour, values and senses of self and identity" (Dupont-Joshua, 2003 p. 66) that are fluid and exposed to the lived reality of people's lives. Understanding culture and difference in this way provides opportunities for partners to develop old, new, or alternative responses to peoples' distress that are culturally embedded and owned.

This proposed framework is based on the idea of praxis—of a theory and practice continuum. Theory comes from clarity of thinking, and without practice (which corrects the theory), there won't be clarity. Through praxis and the participation as equal partners, this framework can release the creative energy of people, from which local understandings and wisdoms can emerge. It can set in motion organic socio-cultural dynamics within each society, which can lead to a new kind of transitional pathway to deal with distress. It could also be the precursor to building new kinds of collaboration that are participatory, pluralist, and truly democratic. This support system also helps in the further multiplication of the process in a non-alienating manner, in contrast to the biomedical model of "expert" and "amateur". This too can promote a new kind of research collaboration for both insiders and outsiders; and a transparent system for freely communicating knowledge within the micro-level processes to provide a countervailing force. In other words, this framework encourages a better sharing of power, a better balance between the outsiders and insiders, and of course between people and nature.

Context in this framework is a very important dimension. As the collaboration can happen between two individuals, communities, or professional research, it is paramount to understand the social, political, cultural, economic, and environmental context of the collaboration. Further, there can be circumstantial context, which could be individual or group dynamics, spirituality, and intersectional conditions such as physical disabilities, and unforeseen circumstances. Although we have presented these contexts separately in Fig. 6.1, they all are interconnected and contribute to the collaborative efforts in different levels. The outsiders must learn the context while insiders must be mindful about the influences of these contextual impacts.

This framework sets out tasks which are intended both to reverse past processes and to move through a transition to improve wellbeing. This cannot be planned through conventional top-down planning and linear methodologies, which are too prescriptive. In dealing with an open and transparent system, which is complex, chaotic, and unpredictable, there needs to be a great deal of flexibility. There will be targets, but not fixed in a rigid project-oriented manner. There is a continuum of self-corrective activities with in-built monitoring and evaluation. Progress is not in a linear fashion, there is forward momentum and setbacks with conflicts. However, the praxis (action-reflection-action process) based on shared values, and the total knowledge system, operates until the goals are achieved. This is how people's knowledge becomes people's power, and this in turn influences wellbeing.

It is important to revisit an ancient concept, which is important in implementing this proposed framework (Fig. 6.1). This concept can be understood in most ancient philosophies from Hindu, Buddhist, Tao, *Ubuntu*, and Mayan traditions that the human sensory organs are limited in understanding the wonders of this planet or universe. In that understanding, there was a perspective that nothing can be explained in its real form. Lao Tzu, the author of Tao Te Ching from Tao philosophical tradition in the Book 1, Verse 1 (quoted in Le Guin, 1998, p. 3) explained the following:

> The way you can go isn't the real way.
> The name you can say isn't the real name.
>
> Heaven and earth begin in the unnamed.
> Name's the mother of the ten thousand things.
>
> So, the unwanting soul sees what's hidden,
> and the ever-wanting soul sees only what it wants.
>
> Two things, one origin, but different in name, whose identity is mystery.
> Mystery of all mysteries! The door to the hidden.
>
> Lao Tzu, from Tao Te Ching, Book 1, Verse 1
> (Le Guin, 1998, p. 3)

This understanding or realisation that we may be wrong is the first step is to overcoming ignorance. Most problems, including conflicts and wars in this world arise from the attitude that "*I am right!*" The moment one thinks that they are right, that means someone, or others must be wrong.

If everyone thinks that their way is the only right way, that gives rise to conflict. What the ancient philosophies realised was that they can only explain something, and that that explanation may not be the complete and the only truth. This dissecting of good and bad, right, and wrong, and moral and immoral that derives from linear analysis of logical reasoning has made many positive contributions to the human civilization, however, it has also created so many ways to discriminate and destruct. What we argue is that there are many ways to explain the same phenomena or object. In that, we argue that no one perspective is entirely correct. This is the prime time to change the linear thinking of biomedical sciences with its reductionist attitude and to open our minds to learn from different epistemologies.

6.6 An Explanation

It is important for us to provide a final explanation for this framework that we are proposing (Fig. 6.1). By no means do we argue that this is "the" way forward. There are many different ways to achieve a collaboration and to create new models beyond the capital marketplace. Many scholars and activists such as Mignolo (2009), Kleinman (2006), Sen (1999), and Illich (1973) have provided different models and frameworks. Further, this is not a "universal" model, but a framework that can be adapted in different contexts. And since any adaptation that is reached will be as an agreement between insiders and outsiders, this can itself bring new elements to the framework and opens the door to variations and even new additions or rejections to what is proposed here. Finally, this is not strictly a framework for mental health and wellbeing. This framework derives from the same idea that everything and everyone is interconnected. Mental health and wellbeing cannot be facilitated without physical, social, and spiritual health and wellbeing. Overall health cannot be facilitated without people-owned development and strong connections to nature and natural processes.

Let us conclude this chapter from an *Umunthu* perspective. The wellbeing of the individual is intertwined with the collective wellbeing of the family, community, and society at large. This framework attempts to facilitate that. Central to *Umunthu* philosophy is that inherent dignity and worth of every individual, which encourages and facilitates empathy, compassion, and a sense of responsibility towards each other. This is the inclusivity, and cooperation that is needed in collaborations. *Umunthu* teaches that individual mental health and wellbeing cannot be achieved in isolation but from fostering harmonious relationships and contributing to the welfare of everyone. This is the opposite of the capital marketplace that promotes isolation, competition, and the relentless pursuit of individual gain, which in return brings distress, unhappiness, sadness, and frustration. In an *Umunthu* approach, self-advancement means collaboration, social cohesion, and contributes to the improvement of collective wellbeing.

References

Angermeyer, M. C., Holzinger, A., Carta, M. G., & Schomerus, G. (2011). Biogenetic explanations and public acceptance of mental illness: Systematic review of population studies. *The British Journal of Psychiatry: the Journal of Mental Science, 199*(5), 367–372.

Bayetti, C., Bakhshi, P., Davar, B., Khemka, G. C., Kothari, P., Kumar, M., Kwon, W., Mathias, K., Mills, C., Montenegro, C. R., Trani, J. F., & Jain, S. (2023). Critical reflections on the concept and impact of "scaling up" in global mental health. *Transcultural Psychiatry, 60*(3), 602–609.

Breen, L. J. (2021). Harnessing social support for bereavement now and beyond the COVID-19 pandemic, editorial. *Palliative Care and Social Practice, 15.*

Burgess, R., & Mathias, K. (2017). Community mental health competencies: A new vision for global mental health. In R. G. White, S. Jain, D. M. Orr, & U. M. Read (Eds.), *The Palgrave handbook of sociocultural perspectives on global mental health.* Palgrave Macmillan.

Burgess, R. A., Jain, S., Pederson, I., & Lund, C. (2019). Social interventions: A new era for global mental health? *Lancet Psychiatry Online.* https://doi.org/10.1016/S2215-0366(19)30397-9

Butterfly Peace Garden. (2000). *Green paper: Towards a foreign policy for the democratic anarchy of the butterfly peace garden of Batticaloa.* BPG.

Campbell, C., & Burgess, R. (2012). The role of communities in advancing the goals of the movement for global mental health. *Transcultural Psychiatry, 49*(3–4), 379–395.

Cox, N., & Webb, L. (2015). Poles apart: Does the export of mental health expertise from the global north to the global south represent a neutral relocation of knowledge and practice? *Sociology of Health & Illness, 37*(5), 683–697.

Di Gessa, G., Maddock, J., Green, M. J., Thompson, E. J., McElroy, E., Davies, H. L., Mundy, J., Stevenson, A. J., Kwong, A. S., Griffith, G. J., & Katikireddi, S. V. (2022). Pre-pandemic mental health and disruptions to healthcare, economic and housing outcomes during the COVID-19 pandemic: Evidence from 12 UK longitudinal studies. *The British Journal of Psychiatry, 220*(1), 21–30.

Dupont-Joshua, A. (Ed.). (2003). *Working inter-culturally in counselling settings.* Brunner-Routledge.

Eyre, A. (2019). The value of peer support groups following disaster: From Aberfan to Manchester. *Bereavement Care, 38*(2–3), 115–121.

Fernando, S. (2014). *Mental health worldwide: Culture, globalization and development.* Palgrave Macmillan.

Fricker, M. (2007). *Epistemic injustice: Power and the ethics of knowing.* Oxford University Press.

Friedman, K. S. (2003). *Myths of the free market.* Algora Publishing.

Halliburton, M. (2023). Hegemony versus pluralism: Ayurveda and the movement for global mental health. *Anthropology & Medicine, 30*(2), 85–102.

Heap, C. J., Jennings, H. M., Mathias, K., et al. (2022). Participatory mental health interventions in low-income and middle-income countries: A realist review protocol. *BMJ Open, 12*, e057530.

Hengartner, M. P. (2017). Methodological flaws, conflicts of interest, and scientific fallacies: Implications for the evaluation of Antidepressants' efficacy and harm. *Frontiers in Psychiatry, 8*, 275.

Illich, I. (1973). *Tools of conviviality.* Harper & Row Publishers.

Jayawickrama, J. (2010). *Rethinking mental health and wellbeing interventions in disaster and conflict affected communities: Case studies from Sri Lanka, Sudan and Malawi.* Doctoral dissertation, Northumbria University.

Jordan, L. S., Seponski, D. M., Kelley, A., & Krpo, N. (2022). The politics of humanitarian aid: A case study of EMDR in Cambodia. *Psychotherapy and Politics International, 20*(1&2), 1–21.

Kirmayer, L. J., & Pedersen, D. (2014). Toward a new architecture for global mental health. *Transcultural Psychiatry, 51*(6), 759–776.

Kleinman, A. (2006). *What really matters: Living a moral life amidst uncertainty and danger.* Oxford University Press.

Korn, L. (1997). *Community trauma and development.* University College, Dublin and the Center for World Indigenous Studies.

Kottai, S. R., & Ranganathan, S. (2020). Task-shifting in community mental health in Kerala: Tensions and ruptures. *Medical Anthropology, 39*(6), 538–552.

Le Guin, U. K. (1998). *Lao Tzu: Tao Te Ching: A book about the way and the power of the way.* Shambhala Publications.

Lund, C. (2017). Balancing the local and the global: Commentary on 'globalizing mental health: Challenges and new visions' section. In R. G. White, S. Jain, D. M. Orr, & U. M. Read (Eds.), *The Palgrave handbook of sociocultural perspectives on global mental health.* Palgrave Macmillan.

Lund, C. (2023). Global mental health and its social determinants: How should we intervene? *Behaviour Research and Therapy, 169*, 104402.

Martín-Baró, I. (1989). Political violence and war as causes of psychosocial trauma in El Salvador. *International Journal of Mental Health, 18*(1), 3–20.

Martín-Baró, I. (1990). War and the psychosocial trauma of Salvadoran children. *Posthumous presentation to American Psychological Association.*

Mathias, K., Singh, P., Butcher, N., Grills, N., Srinivasan, V., & Kermode, M. (2019). Promoting social inclusion for young people affected by psychosocial disability in India – A realist evaluation of a pilot intervention. *Global Public Health, 14*(12), 1718–1732.

Memon, R., Asif, M., Khoso, A. B., Tofique, S., Kiran, T., Chaudhry, N., Husain, N., & Edwards, S. J. (2021). Recognising values and engaging communities across cultures: Towards developing a cultural protocol for researchers. *BMC Medical Ethics, 22*(1), 47.

Mignolo, W. D. (2009). Epistemic disobedience, independent thought and decolonial freedom. *Theory, Culture & Society, 26*(7–8), 159–181.

Mills, C. (2018). From 'invisible problem' to global priority: The inclusion of mental health in the sustainable development goals. *Development and Change, 49*(3), 843–866.

Mills, C., & Fernando, S. (2014). Globalising mental health or pathologising the global south? Mapping the ethics, theory and practice of global mental health. *Disability and the Global South, 1*(2), 188–202.

Mills, C., & Hilberg, E. (2019). 'Built for expansion': The 'social life' of the WHO's mental health GAP intervention guide. *Sociology of Health and Illness, 41*(S1), 162–175.

Nandakumar, P. (1971). *Kambar Ramayanam. A condensed version in English verse and prose.* Sahitya Akademi.

Nussbaum, M. C. (2011). Capabilities, Entitlements, Rights: Supplementation and Critique. *Journal of Human Development and Capabilities, 12*(1), 23–37.

Oehring, D., & Gunasekera, P. (2024). Ethical frameworks and Global Health: A narrative review of the "leave no one behind" principle. *INQUIRY: The Journal of Health Care Organization, Provision, and Financing, 61.* https://doi.org/10.1177/00469580241288346

Olivier de Sardan, J. P., Diarra, A., & Moha, M. (2017). Travelling models and the challenge of pragmatic contexts and practical norms: The case of maternal health. *Health Research Policy and Systems, 15*(Suppl 1), 60.

Oti, S. O., & Ncayiyana, J. (2021). Decolonising global health: Where are the southern voices? *BMJ Global Health, 6*, e006576.

Patel, V. (2014). Rethinking mental health care: Bridging the credibility gap. *Intervention, 12*(Supplement 1), 15–20.

Percudani, M., Barbui, C., & Tansella, M. (2004). The effect of second-generation antipsychotics on employment and productivity in individuals with schizophrenia: An economic perspective. *PharmacoEconomics, 22*, 701–718.

Perera, C., Salamanca-Sanabria, A., Caballero-Bernal, J., Feldman, L., Hansen, M., Bird, M., Hansen, P., Dinesen, C., Wiedemann, N., & Vallières, F. (2020). No implementation without cultural adaptation: A process for culturally adapting low-intensity psychological interventions in humanitarian settings. *Conflict and Health, 14*, 1–12.

Prashad, V. (2014). *The poorer nations: A possible history of the global south.* Verso Books.

Radhakrishnan, S. (1950). *The dhammapada: With introductory essays, Pali text.* English Translation and Notes. Oxford University Press.

Radhakrishnan, S. (1963). *Bhagavad Gita.* George Allen and Unwin Ltd.

Ridde, V., & Olivier de Sardan, J. P. (2022). The development world: Conflicts of interest at all levels. *Revue internationale des études du développement, 249*, 247–269.

Sashidharan, S. P., White, R., Mezzina, R., Jansen, S., & Gishoma, D. (2016). Global mental health in high-income countries. *The British Journal of Psychiatry, 209*(1), 3–5.

Sefasi, A., Crumlish, N., Samalani, P., Kinsella, A., O'Callaghan, E., & Chilale, H. (2008). A little knowledge: Caregiver burden in schizophrenia in Malawi. *Social Psychiatry and Psychiatric Epidemiology, 43*, 160–164.

Sen, A. (1999). *Development as freedom.* Oxford University Press.

Sinha, B. (2023). *The Bengal famine and cultural production: Signifying colonial trauma.* Routledge.

Sinha, N., & Ranganathan, S. (2020). Living with voices: A thematic analysis of individuals' experiences of voice-hearing in India. *Psychosis, 12*(2), 115–127.

Sood, A. (2016). The global mental health movement and its impact on traditional healing in India: A case study of the Balaji temple in Rajasthan. *Transcultural Psychiatry, 53*(6), 766–782.

Srinivasan, V., Jain, S., Kwon, W., Bayetti, D., Anish, C. V., & Mathias, K. (2023). What innovative practices and processes are used to deliver psychosocial care in India? A qualitative case study of three non-profit community mental health organisations. *SSM – Mental Health, 4*, 100220.

Taylor, K., & Burgess, G. H. (2019). Views of non-Western trainee or recently-qualified practitioner psychologists on the import of Western psychology into their indigenous non-Western cultures. *International Journal of Mental Health, 48*, 272–287.

White, R. G., Gregg, J., Batten, S., Hayes, L. L., & Kasujja, R. (2017). Contextual behavioral science and global mental health: Synergies and opportunities. *Journal of Contextual Behavioral Science, 6*(3), 245–251.

White, R. G., & Sashidharan, S. P. (2014). Towards a more nuanced global mental health. *British Journal of Psychiatry, 204*, 415–417.

Wright, J., Mazumdar, P., Barua, D., Lina, S., Bibi, H., Kanwal, A., Mujeeb, F., Naz, Q., Safi, R., Ul Haq, B., & Rana, R. Z. (2020). Integrating depression care within NCD provision in Bangladesh and Pakistan: A qualitative study. *International Journal of Mental Health Systems, 14*, 1–13.

Wignaraja, P. (1991). *Participatory development: Learning from South Asia*. United Nations University Press.

Wolfe, S., & Vitebsky, P. (2003). Assumptions and expectations: Adapting to diverse cultural settings. In A. Dupont-Joshua (Ed.), *Working inter-culturally in counselling settings*. Brunner-Routledge.

World Health Organisation. (2008). *Task shifting: Global recommendations and guidelines*. WHO.

World Health Organisation. (2010). *mhGAP intervention guide for mental, neurological and substance use disorders in non-specialized health settings*. WHO.

Wright, J., & Jayawickrama, J. (2021). "We need other human beings in order to be human": Examining the indigenous philosophy of Umunthu and strengthening mental health interventions. *Culture, Medicine, and Psychiatry, 45*, 613–628.

Wright, J., & Maliwichi-Senganimalunje, L. (2020). Pluralism and practicality: Village health Workers' responses to contested meanings of mental illness in southern Malawi. *Anthropology & Medicine, 27*(1), 32–48.

CHAPTER 7

Conclusion

7.1 Distress as an Inside Experience

> Normal and shared moral experience of this sort is so troubling precisely because what looks so wrong from outside...may not look that way from the inside.
>
> Kleinman (2006, p. 2).

Throughout this book we have attempted to argue against the 'ethnocentricity' and 'universality' that originates from the Euro-North American context and have shown how this may be seen as an extension of the colonial project. In focusing on this universalist tendency to the narrative of distress, psychological and emotional problems, or mental illness, a number of assumptions have become apparent. In the face of all our attempts to control threats to our wellbeing, whether in Malawi, Sri Lanka, the UK or anywhere else in the world, life is always uncertain and dangerous, and people get distressed and suffer. Kleinman (2006) agrees that these everyday struggles, where we try to hold onto those things that matter most to us, are the stuff of life, and at risk of repeating the point, we argue that even people in a 'rich' country like the UK experience distress based on their class, poverty levels, race, environment, and disasters. However, the assumption that people respond to crises that emerge from uncertainty and dangers in the same way globally is problematic, and Kleinman's

J. Jayawickrama, J. Wright, *Under the Gaze of Global Mental Health*, The Politics of Mental Health and Illness,
https://doi.org/10.1007/978-3-031-78258-9_7

above observation reminds us of that perspectives from outside and from within a culture may be entirely different.

Our social, political, cultural, economic, and environmental contexts, as well as our wisdoms, and traditions, all define our suffering, our levels of distress and responses to it. In that, we invite readers to engage with the materials presented in this book from within your own context. We do not claim that our way is the only way to understand distress, but we are sure that there are many ways, including the biomedical model. What we have argued is that while there is value from the biomedical model, it does not provide all the answers. Such a position renders as problematic experts promoting the MGMH's one explanation and response. What we point out is that this co-option of explanation and response by movements like the MGMH is a form of coloniality—a colonisation of the mind.

As we have seen in earlier chapters, colonised people have been forced to suppress their language, ancient wisdoms, and pride to obtain an identity of personhood or community defined by the coloniality of the powerful. Indeed, the success of coloniality has been said to hinge on its effortless reproduction of what is considered superior knowledge (Maldonado-Torres, 2007; Mignolo, 2011). In this way, scientific knowledge systems, including the biomedical model, have come to define what is considered to be human, how to feel, and even what are good emotions, and bad emotions within the culture. Coloniality maintains, and reinforces dominant ways of knowing, thinking, and understanding. In many cultures such as in Malawi and Sri Lanka, how we make sense of the world extends beyond body-bound senses. Such understandings reach beyond the Euro-North American biomedical model and, whether such ideas are rejected or accepted, they remain credible sources of wisdom for both understanding and experiencing distress (Farias et al., 2013) and signal a need for responses that are inclusive of different health systems (Ibeneme et al., 2017). Through this book, we invite you to re-examine your own thoughts, mainly to establish clarity. Although, there is a lot of discussion and a push for such critical thinking, what does this mean? The following ancient Buddhist text, which we also presented in Chap. 1, advises on a way to establish a clarity of thought and critical thinking:

> Yes, Kalamas, it is proper that you have doubt, that you have perplexity, for a doubt has arisen in a matter which doubtful. Now, look you Kalamas, do not be led by reports, or traditions, or hearsay. Be not led by the authority of religious texts, nor by mere logic or inference, not by considering

appearances, not by the delight in speculative opinions, nor by the idea: 'this is our teacher.' But O Kalamas, when you know for yourselves that certain things are unwholesome (*akkusala*) and wrong, and bad, then give them up ... And when you know for yourselves that certain things are wholesome (*kusala*) and good, then accept them and follow them.

Rahula, 1990

(Cited in Henning, 2002, pp. 59–60)

When our thoughts are clear, then we can practise. By practising, we become clearer in our thoughts. This is praxis. In that, when we talk about a decolonial praxis, it is about resistance, rebellion, and transgression against coloniality—the coloniality of the mind. In mental health, a decolonial praxis can create space to interrogate the privileges and disadvantages of Euro-North American concepts, especially within the context of power in the coloniality of the capital marketplace. With this in mind, it is important to ask questions, such as who has developed these concepts? What justifies the labels of mental health in my own context? And is this in the best interests of people that are suffering through uncertainty and danger? Privileged experts and researchers need to reflect on what their motivations are for conducting research and programmes in non-European and non-North American societies. We might be able to collaborate with professionals, traditional healers, and medical practitioners in those countries as equal partners. However, it is important to consider that power disparities impact on where the theories, concepts, and frameworks that view the world, originate from. How often do psychiatrists, clinical psychologists, and mental health experts who were trained in Euro-North American contexts, consider spirituality, dreams, imagination, dead ancestors, and intuition in their approaches? Why are we using data and findings as evidence to reaffirm Euro-North American ways of understanding the world while ignoring or diminishing perspectives from the rest of the world? As Kleinman's quote at the start of this chapter reminds us, insider and outsider perspectives naturally differ, and a moral experience can only be properly understood by those from within a cultural group. How erroneous then to assume that such experiences, or the knowledges that inform them, can be judged from an outsider. This remains true when the effectiveness of traditional, indigenous, or even biomedical knowledge is being judged.

So, a holistic and locally informed methodology is essential to understanding people's mental health and responses in different contexts. This means that any single discipline analysis which flows from the biomedical system is insufficient. A few factors singled out from a rich social reality become very abstract. The oppressed become truly oppressed only when they become repressed in the mind, for example, when people do not have access to the source of the knowledge from which they draw strength. As we explained in the book, the biomedical model differentiates "experts" who have knowledge and "people" who are assumed not have knowledge, and that, without the expert help, people cannot figure out how to deal with external challenges to life. To break out of this biomedical thinking which has penetrated the globe, a major "decolonisation of the minds" of scholars and practitioners alike is required. And it is within this context that we present our humble suggestion of a framework for collaboration in the field of health and wellbeing. For our two case studies demonstrate that from the 'outsider perspective', each may appear very different. Sure, from different continents, they are very different contexts. However, from the 'inside' each have very similar struggles in their relationship with biomedicine. In Sri Lanka and Malawi, critique arises out of indigenous philosophical and religious traditions of healing which continue to have contemporary resonance that respond to peoples' heritage, life experiences and challenges. In the UK, the critique of the dominant biomedical agenda derives from social and disability movements, the mental health service-user movements and a few critical health professionals that expose the limitations of explaining social issues as illness. In our experience, what is interesting—and indicative of historical socio-political context—is that in the UK, biomedicine has become the indigenous tradition. Any medical pluralism tends to be imported to the country—for example, acupuncture, homeopathy, chiropractic—and is not indigenous to the UK people. The pre-Christian traditions disappeared with the forceful impact of the Enlightenment period as biomedical scientific thinking dominated the healing landscape. And yet, through colonial and capital power, that indigenous Western European biomedical system achieved a global language and authority, with all its colonist implications, as a result that a common understanding of different continents was arrived at:

> "In Europe they have knowledge, in Africa we have culture!"
> Anu Pillay, a South African Feminist, (2018).[1]

[1] Hailing from South Africa, Dr. Anu Pillay is a global humanitarian and development practitioner, researcher, and academic. She has been collaborating with Janaka for many years, and she mentioned this during the final stage of her doctoral journey in January 2018.

But what does this mean in the discourse of mental health and wellbeing? For we have seen different, but parallel, processes throughout this book. From Malawi, the colonial and postcolonial experiences have highlighted the epistemic injustices and silencing of indigenous knowledge which are grounded in contemporary understandings of mental health and health practices. From Sri Lanka, colonialism has been revisited when Western definitions of trauma have been urged which are "alien" to local concepts and languages. And in the UK, we have seen how a colonial influence across class divides has sought to transform socio-economic problems into mental disorders to be treated.

7.2 Global Mental Health as Coloniality of Power

As we highlighted in Chap. 2, the professionalisation of mental health and wellbeing has divided between knowledge and culture. But this division is problematic since although both knowledge and culture are productions of societies, 'knowledge' attracts more power while 'culture' is seen as "exotic", "traditional", "unscientific" and "romantic". And, as we discussed, it is the globalisation of the capital marketplace that has strengthened this coloniality of knowledge. For globalisation, as we see it, is the result of a process that began with the colonial European-centred capitalism. As argued by Quijano (2000):

> Coloniality is a constituent and a specific element of the pattern of capitalist power. It is based on the imposition of a racial/ethnic classification on the world's population as a cornerstone of the pattern of power and operates in each of the planes, spheres and dimensions, material and subjective, of everyday social existence and societal level.
>
> Quijano (2000, p. 342), quoted in Restrepo (2018, p. 1)

From this context, it might be argued that the facilitation of a power balance is nearly impossible. But this is why it is important to think beyond coloniality, especially from a knowledge perspective. As Dabashi (2013) strongly argues:

> The question of Eurocentricism is now entirely blase'. Of course, Europeans are Eurocentric and see the world from their vantage point, and why should they not? … The question is rather the manner in which non-European

> thinking can reach self-consciousness and evident universality, not at the cost of whatever European philosophers may think of themselves for the world at large, but for the purpose of offering alternative (complementary or contradictory) visions of reality more rooted in the lived experiences of people in Africa, in Asia, in Latin America – countries and climes once under the spell of the thing that calls itself 'the West' but happily no more.

This is why we keep referring to a decolonisation of the mind. From an *Umunthu*, Buddhist, and Hindu philosophical perspective, everyone has the ultimate power to manage their mind. And yet, if the mind is filled with ideas that one knowledge is better than another, then it becomes difficult to treat that 'lesser' knowledge as equal. So here it is important to distinguish 'different' from 'better'. Decolonising the mind means recognising and appreciating that there is 'difference'. In the area of care for mental health and wellbeing this means respecting medical and health pluralism. But decolonising doesn't mean not making judgements over what is seen or experienced as 'better' or 'worse'. It means ensuring that those judgements are not imposed by 'outsiders', but instead are made by 'insiders'. Or, as Sen (1999) would much more eloquently argue, that insiders are provided the capacity to make these choices.

However, it seems that the notion of 'decolonisation' itself is inadequate to describe the complex human activities and interactions associated with colonialism, de-colonialism, and globalisation, as they frequently rely on polarised assumptions that pitch 'traditional' from 'modern' positions. At the same time, and in the same way that cultures are both contemporary and fluid (rather than entrenched or fixed), the knowledges and cultures of different traditions continually rub up against each other, and, as we've seen in previous chapters, interact in an ever evolving, and two-way exchange of ideas and positions. So, in this, two opposites can be true at the same time, and there can be both positive and negative impacts of complex interactions such as globalisation. However, it is the indefensible imbalance created by the coloniality of the capital market system that means that the status and privilege of the Global North dominates the rest of the world. But this is an artefact, not an innate condition. To resist and revolt against this power is a decolonisation of minds, because as long as there is a "belief" that the Euro-North American knowledge may not always be superior, the possibility of decolonisation is there.

7.3 A New Beginning

Although the powerful neoliberal political and socio-economic forces that we have described continue to underpin a colonial-type relationship with epistemic injustices, there are indications that the continuance of the original incarnation of an ethnocentric and universalist GMH agenda has become less easy to defend from a health research, clinical and moral standpoint. This becomes apparent, not least, when the biomedical approach displaces people's access to other healing modalities and actively reduces the opportunities for people to gain resolve from their distress (Halliburton, 2023). Two emerging factors appear to be driving this shift.

Firstly, the recognition of the profound impact of 'social determinants' on mental health is becoming a mainstream view in both the Global North and the Global South (Johnson, 2017). In 2019 the UN Special Rapporteur Dainius Pūras' report on mental health reaffirmed the inseparability of mental health outcomes from macro-level social challenges and inequalities (UN OHCHR, 2019). And yet, such assertions will remain simply a rhetoric of mental health policy unless such understandings are translated into the practices of all who seek to promote mental health and wellbeing, whether from inside or outside communities. This is where a second factor of working to optimise local community strengths and ownership of processes that seek to improve health and wellbeing is beginning to gain traction. Facilitation in this way is achieved only through the establishment of relations respectful of historical, socio-cultural contexts and mindful of local priorities and lived realities. This is where allegiance to a set of values and behaviours, such as those embodied in our framework, or from other approaches that establish equal collaborations based on trust, respect, and a shared humanity, becomes vital to address the reality of peoples' lives and suffering. Burgess et al. (2020) have expressed this crucial link:

> The time has come for the global mental health movement to acknowledge the importance of the socio-structural determinants of mental distress, and work alongside communities and policy makers in their efforts to address them.
> Burgess et al. (2020, p. 118).

Srinivasan et al. (2023) too, stress the similar importance that organisations incorporate reflexive practice and two-way flows of knowledge to enable them to address the complex social determinants of mental health.

Again, to engage with communities on such a basis where relational and epistemic powers are shared represents a promising ideological shift to a decolonising agenda.

In fact the sheer weight of research evidence and critique over the past 20 or more years from anthropologists, sociologists, mental health researchers, health practitioners, scholars, activists, people with lived experience of care and caring for people in distress from around the world, a perspective on which we have tried to present in this book, are beginning to show signs that the direction and method of GMH is both challenged and changing. Promisingly too, if change is to be realised, this agitation has been advocated from both outside and from within the MGMH organisation itself. Bemme (2023), for instance, has traced the changes in GMH approach from early conception of technical responses to universal problems through to an emerging construct where local pluralism, multiplicity of approach, fluidity and open-ended practices are all seen as assets rather than liabilities to promoting wellbeing.

The cultural adaptation of GMH interventions, although initially viewed as a rather unnecessary component that delayed and obstructed 'implementation', began to take on more elaborate processes of translation and various layers of validation. Now, however, there is an emerging decolonial recognition that the very attempt to 'adapt' contains assumptions that become harmful cultural appropriations that not only are a derivation from their contextual meaning and far from people's lived experiences, but also retain or even increase the epistemic power of those undertaking the adaptation (Hartmann et al., 2022).

In research too, the move from pursuing a generalisability from scaled-up interventions is beginning to be replaced by more localised research orientations such as realist reviews where the focus is much more on fundamental yet answerable questions like "what works, for whom, where and why?" (Heap et al., 2022). Adopting these localised approaches, usually with grass-roots community organisations, enables the kind of inductive research where the micro interventions that support social aspects of mental health care are illuminated and the detail of such social approaches are exposed (Jain et al., 2024). This offers an exciting and meaningful direction where 'outsiders' work alongside and in equal partnership with insiders in its mission.

Undertaking this shift towards a decolonised approach though does not absolve projects from complexity and challenge, and tensions can still emerge or remain, especially where legitimacies of certain knowledges are retained. Logan and Karter (2022), for instance, in their exploration of psychiatrisation across the globe, highlight the nuanced dispute in the Global South where psychosocial disability movements aiming to transform social opportunities and inclusion were thwarted by other activists' demands for access to psychiatric treatments. Such a challenge remains, as the legacy of psychiatrisation of care can only be addressed through active and honest engagement, focusing on the local and establishing a dialogue for insider and outsider collaborations.

A parallel tension of psychiatrisation can be seen in contemporary UK mental health services, where demographic changes, government financial austerity measures, and decisions like leaving the European Union, have led to a shortage in psychiatrists (McCarey et al., 2022). In response, overseas medical recruitment has rocketed, and international medical graduates now make up 44% of psychiatrist trainees (junior doctors) in the UK (GMC, 2019), Ironically, while the increase in ethnic diversity is welcome and is more reflective of the UK population, this has also brought to the UK a workforce perhaps more familiar with the traditional biological view of psychiatric thinking that was originally exported by British colonial medical institutions. Again, these epistemic flows and historic continuities will be influencing the lives of local people today and the enduring influence of psychiatrisation and professional power remains a challenge, and points to the need for a continued vigilance over the preservation of local knowledges and responses.

7.4 A Common Path

This is why the framework we propose has the prerequisites of trust, respect, and a shared humanity for collaboration. When one engages in a process with these prerequisites, then they are engaging in a decolonisation process of their own minds. We understand this first hand through our own collaboration since 2015. We realised that balancing power is not a mathematical equation of dividing this in half. In some instances, Jerome has more power because he has more experience or understanding of something. In other instances, Janaka has more power based on his experiences or understanding of concepts from a different epistemology. As we continue with our collaboration, we realised that we are becoming more and more conscious about this rhythm of sharing power. As we have trust and respect each other, and share a common realisation of humanity, it does not matter who has the power at any given time. There is no nervousness or inferiority in this collaboration. This is the friendship, and in that we both keep changing our worldviews as friends. These are also not new ideas or experiences.

> We need outside help for analysis and understanding of our situation and experience, but not for telling us what we should do.
>
> An outsider who comes with ready-made solutions and advice is worse than useless. He must first understand from us what our questions are, and help us articulate the questions better, and then help us find solutions. Outsiders also have to change.
>
> He alone is a friend who helps us to think about our problems on our own.
>
> (From a dialogue with a facilitator in the Bhoomi Sena Social Movement, Maharashtra, India 1978/79, Wignaraja, 2005, quoted in Jayawickrama (2013, p.39)

This is easier said than done and, as we have explained, working within a capital marketplace makes this a very challenging and difficult task. But we encourage the reader to approach these challenges with thoughtfulness, humility, and optimism. We hope that through our examples and analysis, we have presented a firm basis from which to understand and critique these complex interactions between the individual and their lived experience of the environment. We hope too that our framework for collaboration offers an ethical and practical guide to working in partnership across cultures. In this we have enlisted learning from the many scholars, researchers, practitioners, and people from around the globe who have shed light and are continuing to grapple with these issues and through which we hope to have offered a counter to progressing colonial thinking and practice in the pursuit of all our wellbeing.

Finally, it is important to understand that in a decolonisation of the mind process, the need for GMH—where there is a global reach—becomes less and less relevant. What emerges through local processes remain local, and outsiders may come and learn from them. However, there won't be an agenda to take what works in Sri Lanka to Malawi or to the UK. Through this learning, there will be different adaptations of frameworks, approaches, and tools, but not from just within one dominant discourse.

What we argue throughout this book is that communities that are affected by disasters, conflicts, and uneven development conditions are capable of dealing with uncertainties and dangers of life without outside "expert" help. Although there are levels of mental health and wellbeing challenges that can be visible to an outsider, it takes an insider's view of a community's customs, cultural practices, local knowledge systems and values that, given their resources, can be marshalled to address distress in an informed, sophisticated yet pragmatic manner. A common theme throughout this book is that suffering through uncertainty and danger is a part of human experience and an attribute to the human condition. Along with the cost of poverty, violence, disasters, and other forms of crises, a deep understanding of mental health and wellbeing in uncertainty and danger is little understood. The onset of such uncertainty and danger are sometimes sudden, like the 2004 tsunami in Sri Lanka. At other times they take the form of a continuous trap of suffering like failed development strategies witnessed in Malawi. Even when suffering is not present in such a striking form, there can be slow deterioration of communities through conditions and policies that ruthlessly disrupt the lives of communities, such as in the UK. And all this is complicated by the type of events that take place and the varied ways that communities and individuals perceive and experience their distress. However, in the middle of the worst circumstances, individuals and communities continue with their lives, livelihoods, and hopes, to celebrate and enjoy. This is an achievement beyond everyday life. And is one made richer still by the collaboration of peoples contributing different knowledges to the cause of promoting the mental health and wellbeing of people everywhere.

References

Bemme, D. (2023). Contingent universality: The epistemic politics of global mental health. *Transcultural Psychiatry, 60*(3), 385–399.

Burgess, R. A., Jain, S., Petersen, I., & Lund, C. (2020). Social interventions: A new era for global mental health? *The Lancet Psychiatry, 7*(2), 118–119.

Dabashi, H. (2013). *Can non-Europeans think? What happens with thinkers who operate outside the European philosophical 'pedigree'?* https://www.aljazeera.com/opinions/2013/1/15/can-non-europeans-think/

Farias, M., Underwood, R., & Claridge, G. (2013). Unusual but sound minds: Mental health indicators in spiritual individuals. *British Journal of Psychology (London, England: 1953), 104*(3), 364–381.

General Medical Council. (2019). *The state of medical Education and Practice in the UK: The workforce report.* https://www.gmc-uk.org/about/what-we-do-and-why/data-and-research/the-state-of-medical-education-and-practice-in-the-uk

Halliburton, M. (2023). Hegemony versus pluralism: Ayurveda and the movement for global mental health. *Anthropology & Medicine, 30*(2), 85–102.

Hartmann, W. E., Saint Arnault, D. M., & Gone, J. P. (2022). Conceptualizing culture in (global) mental health: Lessons from an urban American Indian behavioral health clinic. *Social Science & Medicine, 301*, 114899.

Heap, C. J., Jennings, H. M., Mathias, K., Gaire, H., Gumbonzvanda, F., Gumbonzvanda, N., Gupta, G., Jain, S., Maharjan, B., Maharjan, R., Maharjan, S. M., Mahat, P., Pillai, P., Webber, M., Wright, J., & Burgess, R. (2022). Participatory mental health interventions in low-income and middle-income countries: A realist review protocol. *BMJ Open, 12*(4), Article e057530. https://doi.org/10.1136/bmjopen-2021-057530

Henning, D. H. (2002). *A manual for Buddhism and deep Ecology* (Special Ed.). The World Buddhist University.

Ibeneme, S., Eni, G., Ezuma, A., & Fortwengel, G. (2017). Roads to health in developing countries: Understanding the intersection of culture and healing. *Current Therapeutic Research, Clinical and Experimental, 86*, 13–18.

Jain, S., Pillai, P., & Mathias, K. (2024). Opening up the 'black-box': What strategies do community mental health workers use to address the social dimensions of mental health? *Social Psychiatry and Psychiatric Epidemiology*, 1–10.

Jayawickrama, J. (2013). 'If they can't do any good, they shouldn't come': Northern evaluators in southern realities. *Journal of Peacebuilding & Development, 8*(2), 26–41.

Johnson, S. (2017). Social interventions in mental health: A call to action. *Social Psychiatry and Psychiatric Epidemiology, 52*, 245–247.

Kleinman, A. (2006). *What really matters: Living a moral life amidst uncertainty and danger*. Oxford University Press.

Logan, J., & Karter, J. M. (2022). Psychiatrization of resistance: The co-option of consumer, survivor, and ex-patient movements in the global south. *Frontiers in Sociology, 7*, 784390.

Maldonado-Torres, N. (2007). On the coloniality of being: Contributions to the development of a concept. *Cultural Studies, 21*(2–3), 240–270.

McCarey, M., Dayan, M., Jarman, H., Hervey, T., Fahy, N., Bristow, D., & Greer, S. L. (2022). *Health and Brexit: Six years on*. Research Report. Nuffield Trust.

Mignolo, W. (2011). *The darker side of western modernity: Global futures, decolonial options*. Duke University Press.

Quijano, A. (2000). Colonialidad del poder y clasificación social [Coloniality of power and social classification]. *Journal of World-Systems Research, 1*(2), 342–386.

Restrepo, E. (2018). Coloniality of power. *The International Encyclopaedia of Anthropology, 1*, 1–6.

Sen, A. (1999). *Development as freedom*. Oxford University Press.

Srinivasan, V., Jain, S., Kwon, W., Bayetti, C., Cherian, A. V., & Mathias, K. (2023). What innovative practices and processes are used to deliver psychosocial care in India? A qualitative case study of three non-profit community mental health organisations. *SSM-Mental Health, 4*, 100220.

UN OHCHR. (2019, April 12). *Report of the special rapporteur on the right of everyone to the enjoyment of the highest attainable standard of physical and mental health*. https://www.ohchr.org/en/special-procedures/sr-health

Index

J. Jayawickrama, J. Wright, *Under the Gaze of Global Mental Health*, The Politics of Mental Health and Illness,
https://doi.org/10.1007/978-3-031-78258-9

The manufacturer's authorised representative in the EU is Springer Nature Customer Service Centre GmbH, Europaplatz 3, 69115 Heidelberg, Germany. If you have any concerns regarding our products, please contact ProductSafety@springernature.com

Printed and bound by CPI Group (UK) Ltd, Croydon, CR0 4YY
01/10/2026
02225879-0011